Keto Cl
Cookbook

150 EVERYDAY EASY, DELICIOUS AND LOW CARB RECIPES WITH INCREDIBLE TASTE FOR A KETOGENIC DIET. BOOST YOUR METABOLISM AND LIVE WELL EVERY DAY

April R. Brown

Table of Content

SNACKS

DESSERT   111

OTHER KETO CHAFFLES RECIPES — 130

CONCLUSION 183

INTRODUCTION

The new popular food in the keto world is chaffles (short for cheese waffles). It's no surprise— it has a lot to do with the chaffle. A simple recipe for keto is moist, golden brown, free of sugar, low-carb, and very easy to make.

In just a few minutes, you can whip up a basic recipe with only two ingredients eggs and cheese. With a range of sweet and savory choices, you can also customize your chaffle, use it instead of a hamburger bun or bagel, make a chaffle sandwich, or transform it into a pizza chaffle.

This ultimate chaffles + keto chaffle recipe to cover all you need to know, including cheese waffle recipes, nutrition and net carbs, and popular traditional chaffle variations.

A chaffle, or cheese waffle, is an egg and cheese keto waffle. Chaffles become a popular snack of keto / low-carb.

Using a waffle iron or a mini waffle machine, you can prepare a chaffle. the cooking time is just a few minutes, so you end up with a warm, salty, tasty bread / waffle substitute when you cook the chaffle right.

For practitioners of the keto diet, chaffles become a bit of a craze. They are less fussy to make and easy to customize than most keto bread recipes. You can create your own version of the basic recipe for a chaffle, from savory to sweet and anything in between.

You can also change the type of cheese you are using, resulting in major changes in the chaffle's flavor and texture. The two most popular options are cheddar cheese and mozzarella cheese, but you can also add parmesan cheese, cream cheese, or any other cheese that melts well. Chaffles nutrition and Carb count You'll get about half a cup of cheese and two chaffles out of a large egg. Your Calories and net carb count will change a bit based on the cheese you use. As usually, if you're using actual, whole milk cheese such as cheddar or mozzarella (as opposed to cream cheese or American cheese), it's absolutely carb-free.

An average two-chaffle serving size contains roughly:

- 300 Calories

- 0 g gross Carbs

- 0 g net Carbs

- 20 g Protein

- 23 g Fat

As you can see, chaffles are about so keto as a meal can be: high-fat, high-protein, and zero-carb. We still work on the diet of carnivores, as long as you eat cheese.

How to Make Extra Crispy Chaffles There are a few tips you're going to want to know to make your chaffles particularly crispy.

First of all, don't eat the waffle iron directly from your chaffles. At first, they're going to be soggy and eggy, but if you let them stay for 3-4 minutes, they're going to crisp up.

Third, you should add an extra coating of shredded cheddar cheese to both sides of the waffle maker's surface for extra crispy chaffles (or another cheese that gets crispy, like parmesan). Lay down the shredded cheese, pour over the batter, add more cheese, and cook the chaffle normally. You'll end up stuck in the top of the chaffle with crispy brown bits of cheese. Use these two tips to make it easier for the crispest chaffles.

How is it possible to use your chaffles?

There are many popular ways of eating chaffles.

- Clean. Chaffles are perfect as a breakfast meal on their own. In addition to pancakes, sausage, avocado and other regular keto breakfast food, you should feed them.

- Sandwich chaffle keto. Create two chaffles for your dream sandwich and use them as toast. Chaffles are perfect for BLTs, turkey clubs, sandwiches for coffee, or any other keto-friendly snack.

- Desert chaffle. Try one of the sweet variations listed below and serve with your favorite keto ice cream or keto maple syrup.

Traditional Chaffle Recipe variations You can customize your chaffle in all sorts of ways. There are a couple of options here. Cheddar, mozzarella, parmesan, cream cheese — any cheese that spreads well is going to work with a chaffle. Similar cheeses produce different flavors and textures. Try some of them and find your pick.

Use a neutral cheese such as mozzarella or cream cheese, and apply your preferred keto sweetener to the batter before frying it. Whether blueberries or bananas, you can also use chocolate chips or low-sugar foods. For a delicious dessert of the chaffle, finish with keto ice cream or keto whipped cream.

Savory Chaffles Bring to your chaffle savory ingredients such as herbs and spices. Add tomato sauce and extra cheese on top, add oregano, garlic powder and sliced pepperoni in the batter for a pizza chaffle. Or you could use cream cheese to apply all the bagel seasoning for a bagel chaffle to the batter. Serve on top with more cream cheese, capers, onions and smoked salmon. Take the chaffles and come up with your own favorite combinations. These are a great addition to a ketogenic diet and a lot of fun in the kitchen to play with. And check out all of our low-carb recipes for inspiration and more awesome keto food. Ketogenic is a low-carb diet concept (such as the Atkins diet). The aim is to gain more Protein and Fat Calories and less carbohydrate. You cut most of the sugars, including caffeine, coffee, pastries, and white bread, that are easy to digest.

If you eat less than 50 grams of Carbs a day, your body will eventually run out of fuel (blood sugar) that can be used quickly. Usually this takes 3 to 4 days. Then you're going to start breaking down Protein and Fat for nutrition, so you can lose weight. This is what is called ketosis. It is important to note that the ketogenic diet is a short-term diet that focuses on weight loss rather than health benefits.

In the first 3 to 6 months, a ketogenic diet can help you lose more weight than some other diets. This may be because the transformation of Fat into energy requires more Calories than the transformation of carbohydrates into energy. A high-fat, high-Protein diet may also please you better, so you're eating less, but that's not yet confirmed. Typically, the more common ones are not serious: constipation, moderate low blood sugar, or indigestion. Low-carb diets can result in kidney stones or high acid levels in your bloodstream (acidosis) much less often. Other side effects may include headache, weakness, and irritability; bad breath; and fatugue.

BREAKFAST & BRUNCH

1. Taco Chaffles

Preparation Time: 30 minutes

Servings: 1 large chaffles or 2 mini chaffles

INGREDIENTS

Taco filling ingredients

- 1 tsp of chili powder
- 1 tsp of ground cumin
- 1/2 tsp of garlic powder
- 1/2 tsp of cocoa powder
- 1/4 tsp of onion powder
- 1/4 tsp of salt
- 1/12 tsp of smoked paprika
- 1 tbsp of olive oil
- 1/4 of a pound of ground beef or ground turkey
- 1/2 of a cup of cheddar cheese, shredded
- 1/2 an onion
- 1 handful of cilantros, chopped
- 1 lime, cut into wedges
- Hot sauce of your choice

Tools: waffle maker, mini or regular sized, one mixing bowl, measuring cups and tablespoons, spatula, non-stick cooking spray (or butter), taco stand, medium-sized pan, blender, electric beaters, or whisk.

DIRECTIONS

1. Take all of the taco seasonings and mix together in a bowl.

2. Take the olive oil and put it on the medium-sized pan and add your ground beef or turkey. Put it on medium heat.
3. Add all of the taco meat seasonings to the meat.
4. Continue to stir until the meat has browned.
5. Dice the cilantro, lettuce, onions, and limes.
6. Shred the cheese in a bowl.
7. Take the meat off the heat once it is done. Set aside.
8. Follow the classic chaffle recipe.
9. Once the chaffles are done, put them in a taco stand to help them take shape.
10. Fill the chaffles with the meat, cheese, cilantro, lettuce, onions, and limes.
11. Enjoy!

2. Wasabi Chaffles

Preparation Time: 30 minutes

Servings: 1 large chaffles or 2 mini chaffles

INGREDIENTS

- Japanese toppings ingredients
- 1 whole avocado, ripe
- 5 slices of pickled ginger
- 1 tbsp of gluten-free soy sauce
- 1/3 of a cup of edamame
- 1/4 of a cup of japanese pickled vegetables
- 1/2 pound of sushi-grade salmon, sliced
- 1/4 of a tsp of wasabi

Tools: waffle maker, mini or regular sized, one mixing bowl, measuring cups and tablespoons, spatula, non-stick cooking spray (or butter), blender, electric beaters, or whisk.

DIRECTIONS

1. Cut the salmon and avocado into thin slices. Set aside.

2. If the edamame is frozen, boil it in a pot of water until done. Set aside.
3. Follow the classic chaffle recipe.
4. Once the chaffles are done, pour a tablespoon of soy sauce onto the chaffle and then layer the salmon, avocado, edamame, pickled ginger, pickled vegetables, and wasabi.
5. Enjoy!

3. Loaded Chaffle Nachos

Preparation Time: 30 minutes

Servings: 1 large chaffles or 2 mini chaffles

INGREDIENTS

Nacho ingredients

- Taco meat recipe
- 1 whole avocado, ripe
- 1/2 cup of sour cream
- 1/2 of a cup of cheddar cheese, shredded
- 1/2 an onion
- 1 handful of cilantros, chopped
- 1 lime, cut into wedges
- Hot sauce of your choice

Tools: waffle maker, mini or regular sized, one mixing bowl, measuring cups and tablespoons, spatula, non-stick cooking spray (or butter), blender, electric beaters, or whisk.

DIRECTIONS

1. Dice the cilantro, lettuce, onions, and limes.
2. Shred the cheese in a bowl. Melt if desired.
3. Follow instructions for the taco meat recipe.
4. Follow the classic chaffle recipe.
5. Once the chaffles are done, rip them into triangles.

6. Spread the chaffle triangles onto a plate and layer on the sour cream, meat, avocado, onions, cilantro, cheese, and lime.
7. Enjoy!

4. Mozzarella Panini

Preparation Time: 30 minutes

Servings: 1 large chaffle or 2 mini chaffles

INGREDIENTS

Sandwich filling ingredients

- 1 ounce of mozzarella, thinly sliced
- 1 heirloom tomato, thinly sliced
- 1/4 of a cup of pesto
- 2 fresh basil leaves

Tools: waffle maker, mini or regular sized, one mixing bowl, measuring cups and tablespoons, spatula, non-stick cooking spray (or butter), blender, electric beaters, or whisk.

DIRECTIONS

1. Follow the classic chaffle recipe.
2. Once the chaffles are done, lay two side by side.
3. Spread the pesto on one, then layer the mozzarella cheese and tomatoes and sandwich together.

5. Pizza Chaffle

Preparation Time: 30 minutes

Servings: 1 large chaffles or 2 mini chaffles

INGREDIENTS

Pizza topping ingredients

- 1 ounce of mozzarella, thinly sliced
- 1 tsp of italian seasoning
- 1 tbsp of sugar-free pizza sauce
- 4-6 pepperoni slices

Tools: waffle maker, mini or regular sized, one mixing bowl, measuring cups and tablespoons, spatula, non-stick cooking spray (or butter), baking pan, blender, electric beaters, or whisk.

DIRECTIONS

1. Preheat the oven to 350 degrees f and take out a baking pan.
2. Follow the classic chaffle recipe.
3. Once the chaffles are done, lay them on the baking pan.
4. Spread the tomato sauce on one then layer the mozzarella cheese and pepperoni slices.
5. Bake in the oven for 5-10 minutes or until the cheese is melting.
6. Careful! These mini pizzas are hot!
7. Enjoy!

6. Hamburger Chaffle

Preparation Time: 30 minutes

Servings: 1 large chaffles or 2 mini chaffles

INGREDIENTS

Hamburger ingredients

- 1/3-pound ground beef
- 1/2 teaspoon garlic salt
- 2 slices american cheese

- 2-3 dill pickles
- 1 slice of red onion
- 1 handful of lettuce, shredded
- 1 slice of an heirloom tomato

Tools: waffle maker, mini or regular sized, one mixing bowl, measuring cups and tablespoons, spatula, non-stick cooking spray (or butter), saucepan, blender, electric beaters, or whisk.

DIRECTIONS

1. Slice the onions, shred the lettuce, and slice the tomatoes.
2. Take a medium-sized pan and put on medium heat.
3. Take the ground meat and form into patties, roughly the same size as your chaffle maker.
4. Fry the ground meat on the pan until cooked through. Set aside when done.
5. Follow the classic chaffle recipe.
6. Once the chaffles are done, lay two chaffles side by side.
7. Layer on the lettuce, meat, tomatoes, onions, pickles, and any sauces of your choosing.
8. Enjoy!

7. Blt Chaffle

Preparation Time: 30 minutes

Servings: 1 large chaffles or 2 mini chaffles

INGREDIENTS

Blt ingredients

- 1 tbsp of mayonnaise
- 1 handful of lettuce, shredded
- 1 slice of an heirloom tomato
- 2 slices of bacon

Tools: waffle maker, mini or regular sized, one mixing bowl, measuring cups and tablespoons, spatula, non-stick cooking spray (or butter), saucepan, blender, electric beaters, or whisk.

DIRECTIONS

1. Shred the lettuce and slice the tomatoes.
2. Take a medium-sized pan and put on medium heat.
3. Take the bacon and cook until desired texture, chewy or crunchy.
4. Set aside when done.
5. Follow the classic chaffle recipe.
6. Once the chaffles are done, lay two chaffles side by side.
7. Layer on the mayonnaise, bacon, lettuce, and tomatoes.
8. Enjoy!

8. Chicken and Chaffles

Preparation Time: 30 minutes

Servings: 1 large chaffles or 2 mini chaffles

INGREDIENTS

- Classic chaffle recipe or sweet chaffle recipe
- Keto fried chicken ingredients
- 2 boneless skinless chicken thighs
- Oil for frying

Egg wash ingredients

- 2 large eggs, whole
- 2 tbsp of heavy whipping cream
- Keto breading ingredients
- 2/3 cup of blanched almond flour
- 2/3 cup of grated parmesan cheese
- 1 tsp of salt
- 1/2 tsp of black pepper
- 1/2 tsp of paprika

- 1/2 tsp of cayenne

Tools: waffle maker, mini or regular sized, three mixing bowls, measuring cups and tablespoons, spatula, non-stick cooking spray (or butter), pot for frying, blender, electric beaters, or whisk.

DIRECTIONS

1. Pour 1-3 inches of oil into a pot on high heat.
2. Have the oil heat up to 350 degrees f.
3. While the oil is heating, take a bowl and mix the eggs and heavy cream until well mixed. Set aside.
4. Take another bowl and mix together the breading ingredients. Set aside.
5. Take each thawed chicken thigh and cut into 3-4 evenly sized pieces.
6. Dip each chicken slice in the breading, followed by dipping the slice in the egg wash, and then back in the breading again.
7. Make sure each side is evenly coated with breading.
8. Then dip the chicken slices slowly and carefully into the hot oil.
9. Keep the chicken slices in the oil until the slices are a deep brown and cooked through. About 5-7 minutes.
10. Do only a few slices at a time to avoid overcrowding the pot.
11. Follow the classic chaffle recipe.
12. Serve the chaffles and chicken on a plate and add some sugar-free pancake syrup or hot sauce to taste.
13. Enjoy!

9. <u>Lox Bagel Chaffle</u>

Preparation Time: 30 minutes

Servings: 1 large chaffles or 2 mini chaffles

INGREDIENTS

- Classic chaffle recipe or sweet chaffle recipe
- 2 tbsps of everything bagel seasoning

Filling ingredients

- 1 ounce of cream cheese
- 1 beefsteak tomato, thinly sliced
- 4-6 ounces of salmon gravlax
- 1 small shallot, thinly sliced
- Capers
- 1 tbsp of fresh dill

Tools: waffle maker, mini or regular sized, one mixing bowl, measuring cups and tablespoons, spatula, non-stick cooking spray (or butter), blender, electric beaters, or whisk.

DIRECTIONS

1. Slice the tomato and the shallots.
2. Follow the classic chaffle recipe and add the everything bagel seasoning.
3. Once the chaffles are done, sprinkle more everything bagel seasoning onto the tops of both chaffles.
4. Lay two chaffles side by side and layer on the cream cheese, salmon, and shallots.
5. Sprinkle dill and capers and sandwich the two chaffles together.
6. Enjoy!

10. Chicken Sandwich Chaffle

Preparation Time: 30 minutes

Servings: 1 large chaffles or 2 mini chaffles

INGREDIENTS

Classic chaffle recipe

- Chicken salad ingredients
- 1-1/2 cups chicken, cooked and sliced apart
- 3 tbsp red onion, finely chopped
- 1/4 of a cup of celery, finely chopped
- 1 large hard-boiled egg, chopped
- 1 tbsp of dill pickle relish
- 1/2 cup of mayonnaise
- 1/4 tsp of salt
- 1-2 cracks of freshly ground black pepper

Tools: waffle maker, mini or regular sized, three mixing bowls, measuring cups and tablespoons, spatula, non-stick cooking spray (or butter), blender, electric beaters, or whisk.

DIRECTIONS

1. Slice the onions, celery, and hard-boiled egg until finely chopped. Set aside in a mixing bowl.
2. Cut the chicken into small pieces and add to the mixing bowl.
3. Mix the onions, celery, hard-boiled egg, and chicken together until well combined.
4. Add the mayonnaise, dill relish, salt, and pepper to the mixing bowl and mix together until well combined. Set aside.
5. Follow the classic chaffle recipe.
6. Lay two chaffles side by side and layer on the chicken salad.
7. Sandwich together.
8. Enjoy!

11.   Open-Faced Tuna Melt Chaffle

Preparation Time: 30 minutes

Servings: 1 large chaffles or 2 mini chaffles

INGREDIENTS

Classic chaffle recipe

- Tuna salad ingredients
- 1 can of white meat tuna
- 3 tbsp red onion, finely chopped
- 1/4 of a cup of celery, finely chopped
- 1/2 cup of mayonnaise
- 1/4 tsp of salt
- 1-2 cracks of freshly ground black pepper
- 1-2 slices of cheddar cheese

Tools: waffle maker, mini or regular sized, three mixing bowls, measuring cups and tablespoons, spatula, non-stick cooking spray (or butter), baking sheet, blender, electric beaters, or whisk.

DIRECTIONS

1. Preheat your oven to 350 degrees f.
2. Slice the onions and celery until finely chopped. Set aside in a mixing bowl.
3. Add the tuna to the mixing bowl.
4. Mix the onions, celery, and tuna together until well combined.
5. Add the mayonnaise, salt, and pepper to the mixing bowl and mix together until well combined. Set aside.
6. Follow the classic chaffle recipe.
7. Lay the chaffles side by side on a baking sheet and layer on the tuna salad.
8. Add 1-2 slices of cheese per chaffle.
9. Place in the oven until the cheese is melted.
10. Take out and enjoy immediately.

12.   Hot Dog Chaffle

Preparation Time: 30 minutes

Servings: 1 large chaffles or 2 mini chaffles

INGREDIENTS

- Classic chaffle recipe
- Hot dog ingredients
- 1-2 hot dogs of your choice
- Mustard, ketchup and relish to taste

Tools: waffle maker, mini or regular sized, three mixing bowls, measuring cups and tablespoons, spatula, non-stick cooking spray (or butter), taco stand, baking sheet, blender, electric beaters, or whisk.

DIRECTIONS

1. Cook your hot dogs as you normally would. Either on a grill or in the oven until done.
2. Follow the classic chaffle recipe.
3. Take each chaffle and put in a taco stand to hold shape.
4. Stick a hot dog in each chaffle and top with any added sauce of your choosing.

13.   Cuban Sandwich Chaffle

Preparation Time: 30 minutes

Servings: 1 large chaffles or 2 mini chaffles

INGREDIENTS

- Classic chaffle recipe
- Cubano ingredients
- 1/4 of a pound of ham, cooked and sliced
- 1/4 of a pound of pork, roasted and sliced
- 1/4-pound swiss cheese, thinly sliced
- 3 dill pickles, sliced in half

Tools: waffle maker, mini or regular sized, three mixing bowls, measuring cups and tablespoons, spatula, non-stick cooking spray (or butter), baking sheet, blender, electric beaters, or whisk.

DIRECTIONS

1. Follow the classic chaffle recipe.
2. Take two chaffles and lay side by side.
3. Lay on the meat, cheese, and pickles.
4. Sandwich the two chaffles together.
5. Put the sandwich in a toaster oven if you want it hot.
6. Heat for 5 minutes or until cheese is melted.

14.   Reuben Sandwich Chaffle

Preparation Time: 30 minutes

Servings: 1 large chaffles or 2 mini chaffles

INGREDIENTS

- Classic chaffle recipe

Reuben ingredients

- 1 tbsp of butter (softened)
- 2 tbsp of thousand island dressing with no sugar
- 2 ounces of corned beef, sliced
- 1 ounce of sauerkraut
- 1 ounce of swiss cheese, sliced

Tools: waffle maker, mini or regular sized, three mixing bowls, measuring cups and tablespoons, spatula, non-stick cooking spray (or butter), baking sheet, blender, electric beaters, or whisk.

DIRECTIONS

Follow the classic chaffle recipe.

- Take two chaffles and lay side by side.

- Lay on the thousand island dressing, butter, meat, cheese, and sauerkraut.
- Sandwich the two chaffles together.
- Put the sandwich in a toaster oven if you want it hot.
- Heat for 5 minutes or until cheese is melted.

15. Philly Cheesesteak Chaffle

Preparation Time: 30 minutes

Servings: 1 large chaffles or 2 mini chaffles

INGREDIENTS

Classic chaffle recipe

Philly cheesesteak fillings ingredients

- 1/2 pound of strip loin, trimmed
- 1 tbsp of butter
- 1/2 cup of mushrooms, chopped
- 1/2 cup of onions, thinly sliced
- 1/2 cup of cubano peppers, thinly sliced
- 1/2 cup of poblano peppers, thinly sliced
- 1/2 cup of provolone, sliced

Tools: waffle maker, mini or regular sized, one mixing bowl, measuring cups and tablespoons, spatula, non-stick cooking spray (or butter), two frying pans, blender, electric beaters, or whisk.

DIRECTIONS

1. Chop the onions, peppers, and mushrooms.
2. Slice the provolone. Set aside.
3. Take a frying pan and put it on high heat, add the butter and all of the chopped vegetables. Turn the pan down to medium heat and stir every few minutes until cooked down and caramelized. Set aside.

4. Take another frying pan and cook the trimmed strip loin on medium heat until cooked through. Set aside.
5. Follow the classic chaffle recipe.
6. Take two chaffles and lay side by side.
7. Lay on the meat, onions, peppers, cheese, and mushrooms.
8. Sandwich the two chaffles together.
9. Put the sandwich in a toaster oven if you want it hot.
10. Heat for 5 minutes or until cheese is melted.
11. Enjoy!

16.   Breakfast of Champions Chaffle

Preparation Time: 40 minutes

Servings: 1 large chaffles or 2 mini chaffles

INGREDIENTS

Classic chaffle recipe

- 3 links of your favorite sausage
- 2 whole eggs, for frying
- Salt and pepper to taste
- Hot sauce

Tools: Waffle maker, mini or regular sized, one mixing bowl, measuring cups and tablespoons, spatula, non-stick cooking spray (or butter), frying pan, blender, electric beaters, or whisk.

DIRECTIONS

1. Put a frying pan on medium heat. Once hot, add sausages and cook until brown.
2. Take the sausages out of the pan and fry or scramble your eggs in the sausage grease.
3. Follow the classic chaffle recipe.
4. Once cooled, slice the sausages into circles.
5. Take two chaffles and lay side by side. Add the eggs and sausage and sandwich together.

17.   Steak and Eggs Chaffle

Preparation Time: 40 minutes

Servings: 1 large chaffles or 2 mini chaffles

INGREDIENTS

Classic chaffle recipe

- 1 tbsp of butter
- Quarter pound of sirloin steak
- 2 large eggs, for frying
- Salt and pepper to taste

Tools: waffle maker, mini or regular sized, one mixing bowl, measuring cups and tablespoons, spatula, non-stick cooking spray (or butter), frying pan, blender, electric beaters, or whisk.

DIRECTIONS

1. Put a frying pan on medium heat. Once hot, add the sirloin steak and butter.
2. Cook until brown, about 4-6 minutes per side.
3. Take the steak out of the pan and fry eggs in the grease.
4. Follow the classic chaffle recipe.
5. Once cooled, slice the steak into strips.
6. Take a chaffles and layer on the eggs and steak for an open-faced sandwich.

18.   Fish and Chaffles

Preparation Time: 30 minutes

Servings: 1 large chaffles or 2 mini chaffles

INGREDIENTS

- Classic chaffle recipe or sweet chaffle recipe
- 3/4 of a pound of cod

- Batter from the chicken and chaffles recipe
- Aioli recipe

Tools: waffle maker, mini or regular sized, three mixing bowls, measuring cups and tablespoons, spatula, non-stick cooking spray (or butter), pot for frying, blender, electric beaters, or whisk.

DIRECTIONS

1. Follow the chicken and chaffles recipe, but replace the chicken with cod.
2. Follow the classic chaffle recipe.
3. Follow the aioli recipe.
4. Serve the chaffles and fish on a plate.
5. Enjoy!

19.   Sloppy Joe Chaffles

Preparation Time: 45 minutes

Servings: 1 large chaffles or 2 mini chaffles

INGREDIENTS

Classic chaffle recipe or sweet chaffle recipe

- 1 pound of ground beef or ground turkey
- 1/2 a yellow onion, finely chopped
- 1/3 a red bell pepper, finely chopped
- 1-1/2 cups of sugar free ketchup
- 2 tsp of yellow mustard
- 1 tbsp of swerve brown sweetener
- 1 tsp ground black pepper
- 1 tsp garlic powder
- Salt to taste

Tools: waffle maker, mini or regular sized, three mixing bowls, measuring cups and tablespoons, spatula, non-stick cooking spray (or butter), pot for frying, blender, electric beaters, or whisk.

DIRECTIONS

1. Chop the onions and peppers until fine. Put in a bowl.
2. Put a saucepan on medium heat and add butter to the pan.
3. Once melted, add the onions, peppers, ground meat, and spies on medium heat until the meat browns. 10 minutes.
4. Drain the excess liquid from the saucepan.
5. Mix in the ketchup, mustard, and sweetener until well combined. Cook for another 5 minutes.
6. Transfer the meat into a bowl.
7. Follow the classic chaffle recipe.
8. Take two chaffles and lay them side by side. Pour the sloppy joe's meat onto one and sandwich the chaffles together.

20. Mushroom Sauce

Preparation Time: 40 minutes
Servings: 1 large chaffles or 2 mini chaffles

INGREDIENTS
Classic chaffle recipe or sweet chaffle recipe

- 4 ounces of brown mushrooms, sliced
- 1 shallot, finely chopped
- 1 tbsp of butter
- 1 tbsp of worcestershire sauce
- 1/2 cup of heavy cream
- 1/2 cup of brandy
- Salt and pepper to taste

Tools: waffle maker, mini or regular sized, three mixing bowls, measuring cups and tablespoons, spatula, non-stick cooking spray (or butter), saucepan, blender, electric beaters, or whisk.

DIRECTIONS

1. Chop the shallots and slice the mushrooms.
2. In a saucepan, put on medium heat and sauté the shallots in butter until translucent.
3. Add the mushrooms and cook until brown.
4. Add the brandy and cook until it has evaporated. 5 minutes.
5. Add the cream and worcestershire sauce. Bring to a simmer until the sauce has thickened.
6. Add salt and pepper.
7. Take off heat.
8. Follow the classic chaffle recipe.
9. Take a chaffle and ladle the sauce on top of the chaffle.

21. Turkey Sandwich Chaffle

Preparation Time: 35 minutes
Servings: 1 large chaffles or 2 mini chaffles

INGREDIENTS

- Classic chaffle recipe or sweet chaffle recipe
- 3 slices of pre-sliced turkey
- 2 pieces of lettuce, ripped
- 1 heirloom tomato, sliced
- 1 red onion, thinly sliced into circles
- Aioli recipe

Tools: waffle maker, mini or regular sized, three mixing bowls, measuring cups and tablespoons, spatula, non-stick cooking spray (or butter), saucepan, blender, electric beaters, or whisk.

DIRECTIONS

1. Follow the aioli recipe.
2. Thinly slice the onions but keep them as circles.
3. Slice the tomato also in circle form.
4. Tear the lettuce into the same size as your chaffles.
5. Follow the classic chaffle recipe.

6. Take two chaffles and spread the aioli into one. Layer the lettuce, turkey, tomato, and onions onto

BASIC CHAFFLES

22. Chaffle Mini Sandwich

Preparation Time: 5 min

Cooking Time: 10 min

Servings: 2

INGREDIENTS

- 1 large egg
- 1/8 cup almond flour
- 1/2 tsp. Garlic powder
- 3/4 tsp. Baking powder
- 1/2 cup shredded cheese
- Sandwich filling
- 2 slices deli ham
- 2 slices tomatoes
- 1 slice cheddar cheese

DIRECTIONS

1. Grease your square waffle maker and preheat it on medium heat.
2. Mix together chaffle ingredients in a mixing bowl until well combined.
3. Pour batter intoa square waffle and make two chaffles.
4. Once chaffles are cooked, remove from the maker.
5. For a sandwich,arrange deli ham, tomato slice and cheddar cheese between two chaffles.
6. Cut sandwich from the center.
7. Servings and enjoy!

NUTRITION: Calories: 239 kcal Fats17.86 g Protein17 g Net carbs0.95 g Fiber0.3 g Starch0 g

23.   Chaffles With Topping

Preparation Time: 5 min

Cooking Time: 10 min

Servings: 3

INGREDIENTS

- 1 large egg
- 1 tbsp. Almond flour
- 1 tbsp. Full-Fat greek yogurt
- 1/8 tsp baking powder
- 1/4 cup shredded swiss cheese

Topping

- 4oz. Grillprawns
- 4 oz. Steamed cauliflower mash
- 1/2 zucchini sliced
- 3 lettuce leaves
- 1 tomato, sliced
- 1 tbsp. Flax seeds

DIRECTIONS

1. Make 3 chaffles with the given chaffles ingredients.
2. For serving, arrange lettuce leaves on each chaffle.
3. Top with zucchini slice, grill prawns, cauliflower mash and a tomato slice.
4. Drizzle flax seeds on top.
5. Servings and enjoy!

NUTRITION: Calories: 158 kcal Fats8.41 g Protein17.31 g Net carbs1.14 g Fiber1.1 g Starch0 g

24. Grill Beefsteak and Chaffle

Preparation Time: 5 min

Cooking Time: 10 min

Servings: 1

INGREDIENTS

- 1 beefsteak rib eye
- 1 tsp salt
- 1 tsp pepper
- 1 tbsp. Lime juice
- 1 tsp garlic

DIRECTIONS

1. Prepare your grill for direct heat.
2. Mix together all spices and rub over beefsteak evenly.
3. Place the beef on the grill rack over medium heat.
4. Cover and cook steak for about6 to 8 minutes. Flip and cook for another 4-5 minutes until cooked through.
5. Servings with keto simple chaffle and enjoy!

NUTRITION: Calories: 538 kcal Fats26.97 g Protein68.89 g Net carbs3.07 g Fiber0.8 g Starch0 g

25. Chaffle Cheese Sandwich

Preparation Time: 5 min

Cooking Time: 10 min

Servings: 1

INGREDIENTS

- 2 square keto chaffle

- 2 slice cheddar cheese
- 2 lettuce leaves

DIRECTIONS

1. Prepare your oven on 4000 f.
2. Arrange lettuce leave and cheese slice between chaffles.
3. Bake in the preheated oven for about 4-5 minutes until cheese is melted.
4. Once the cheese is melted, remove from the oven.
5. Servings and enjoy!

NUTRITION: Calories: 215 kcal Fats16.69 g Protein14.42 g Net carbs1.28 g Fiber0.1 g Starch0 g

26. Chaffle Egg Sandwich

Preparation Time: 5 min

Cooking Time: 10 min

Servings: 2

INGREDIENTS

- 2 mini keto chaffle
- 2 slice cheddar cheese
- 1 egg simple omelet

DIRECTIONS

1. Prepare your oven on 4000 f.
2. Arrange egg omelet and cheese slice between chaffles.
3. Bake in the preheated oven for about 4-5 minutes until cheese is melted.
4. Once the cheese is melted, remove from the oven.
5. Servings and enjoy!

NUTRITION: Calories: 495 kcal Fats37.65 g Protein34.41 g Net carbs2.59 g Fiber0.2 g Starch0.01 g

27.   Cauliflower chaffle

Preparation Time: 15 minutes

Servings: 2

INGREDIENTS

- 1 egg, lightly beaten
- 1 cup cauliflower rice
- 1/2 cup parmesan cheese, shredded
- 1/2 cup mozzarella cheese, shredded
- 1 tsp italian seasoning
- 1/4 tsp garlic powder
- 1/4 tsp pepper
- 1/4 tsp salt

DIRECTIONS

1. Preheat your waffle maker.
2. Add all ingredients into the blender and blend until smooth.
3. Spray waffle maker with cooking spray.
4. Pour half batter in the hot waffle maker and cook for 4-5 minutes. Repeat with the remaining batter.
5. Servings and enjoy.

NUTRITION: Calories 239 Fat 15.1 g Carbohydrates 5.1 g Sugar 1.7 g Protein 21 g Cholesterol 116 mg

28.   Perfect Jalapeno Chaffle

Preparation Time: 20 minutes

Servings: 6

INGREDIENTS

- 3 eggs

- 1 cup cheddar cheese, shredded
- 8 oz cream cheese
- 2 jalapeno peppers, diced
- 4 bacon slices, cooked and crumbled
- 1/2 tsp baking powder
- 3 tbsp coconut flour
- 1/4 tsp sea salt

DIRECTIONS

1. Preheat your waffle maker.
2. In a small bowl, mix coconut flour, baking powder, and salt.
3. In a medium bowl, beat cream cheese using a hand mixer until fluffy.
4. In a large bowl, beat eggs until fluffy.
5. Add cheddar cheese and half cup cream in eggs and beat until well combined.
6. Add coconut flour mixture to egg mixture and mix until combined.
7. Add jalapeno pepper and stir well.
8. Spray waffle maker with cooking spray.
9. Pour 1/4 cup batter in the hot waffle maker and cook for 4-5 minutes. Repeat with the remaining batter.
10. Once chaffle is slightly cool then top with remaining cream cheese and bacon.
11. Servings and enjoy.

NUTRITION: Calories 340 Fat 28 g Carbohydrates 6.2 g Sugar 1 g Protein 16.1 g Cholesterol 157 mg

29. Crunchy Zucchini Chaffle

Preparation Time: 20 minutes

Servings: 8

INGREDIENTS

- 2 eggs, lightly beaten

- 1 garlic clove, minced
- 1 1/2 tbsp onion, minced
- 1 cup cheddar cheese, grated
- 1 small zucchini, grated and squeeze out all liquid

DIRECTIONS

1. Preheat your waffle maker.
2. In a bowl, mix eggs, garlic, onion, zucchini, and cheese until well combined.
3. Spray waffle maker with cooking spray.
4. Pour 1/4 cup batter in the hot waffle maker and cook for 5 minutes or until golden brown. Repeat with the remaining batter.
5. Servings and enjoy.

NUTRITION: Calories 76 Fat 5.8 g Carbohydrates 1.1 g Sugar 0.5 g Protein 5.1 g Cholesterol 56 mg

30.   Simple Cheese Bacon Chaffles

Preparation Time: 15 minutes

Servings: 4

INGREDIENTS

- 2 eggs, lightly beaten
- 1/4 tsp garlic powder
- 2 bacon slices, cooked and chopped
- 3/4 cup cheddar cheese, shredded

DIRECTIONS

1. Preheat your mini waffle maker and spray with cooking spray.
2. In a bowl, mix eggs, garlic powder, bacon, and cheese.
3. Pour 2 tbsp of the batter in the hot waffle maker and cook for 2-3 minutes or until set. Repeat with the remaining batter.

4. Servings and enjoy.

NUTRITION: Calories 169 Fat 13.2 g Carbohydrates 0.7 g Sugar 0.3 g Protein 11.6 g Cholesterol 115 mg

31. Cheddar Cauliflower Chaffle

Preparation Time: 13 minutes

Servings: 1

INGREDIENTS

- 1 egg, lightly beaten
- 1 tbsp almond flour
- 1/4 cup cheddar cheese, shredded
- 1/2 cup cauliflower rice
- Pepper
- Salt

DIRECTIONS

1. Preheat your waffle maker.
2. Add all ingredients into the bowl and mix until well combined.
3. Spray waffle maker with cooking spray.
4. Pour batter in the hot waffle maker and cook for 8 minutes or until golden brown.
5. Servings and enjoy.

NUTRITION: Calories 230 Fat 17.3 g Carbohydrates 4.9 g Sugar 1.9 g Protein 15.1 g Cholesterol 193 mg

32. Keto Breakfast Chaffle

Preparation Time: 15 minutes

Servings: 2

INGREDIENTS

- 1 egg, lightly beaten
- ½ cup mozzarella cheese, shredded
- ½ tsp psyllium husk powder
- ¼ tsp garlic powder

DIRECTIONS

1. Preheat your waffle maker.
2. Whisk egg in a bowl with remaining ingredients until well combined.
3. Spray waffle maker with cooking spray.
4. Pour 1/2 of batter in the hot waffle maker and cook until golden brown. Repeat with the remaining batter.
5. Servings and enjoy.

NUTRITION: Calories 55 Fat 3.4 g Carbohydrates 1.3 g Sugar 0.3 g Protein 4.8 g Cholesterol 86 mg

33.   Perfect Keto Chaffle

Preparation Time: 15 minutes

Servings: 2

INGREDIENTS

- 2 eggs, lightly beaten
- 1/2 cup mozzarella cheese, shredded
- 1/2 cup cheddar cheese, shredded
- 1/4 tsp baking powder, gluten-free
- 1 tbsp almond flour
- 1/4 tsp cinnamon
- 1/4 tsp red chili flakes
- 1/4 tsp salt

DIRECTIONS

1. Preheat your waffle maker and spray with cooking spray.
2. In a bowl, whisk eggs with baking powder, almond flour, and salt.
3. Add remaining ingredients and mix until well combined.
4. Pour half of the batter in the hot waffle maker and cook for 3-5 minutes or until golden brown. Repeat with the remaining batter.
5. Servings and enjoy.

NUTRITION: Calories 218 Fat 16.7 g Carbohydrates 2.2 g Sugar 0.6 g Protein 15.3 g Cholesterol 197 mg

34. <u>Cabbage chaffle</u>

Preparation Time: 15 minutes

Servings: 2

INGREDIENTS

- 1 egg, lightly beaten
- 1/3 cup mozzarella cheese, grated
- ½ bacon slice, chopped
- 1 ½ tbsp green onion, sliced
- 2 tbsp cabbage, chopped
- 2 tbsp almond flour
- Pepper
- Salt

DIRECTIONS

1. Add all ingredients in a bowl and stir to combine.
2. Spray waffle maker with cooking spray.
3. Pour half of the batter in the hot waffle maker and cook until golden brown. Repeat with the remaining batter.
4. Servings and enjoy.

NUTRITION: Calories 113 Fat 8.5 g Carbohydrates 2.5 g Sugar 0.7 g Protein 7.5 g Cholesterol 90 mg

35. Simple ham chaffle

Preparation Time: 15 minutes

Servings: 2

INGREDIENTS

- 1 egg, lightly beaten
- 1/4 cup ham, chopped
- 1/2 cup cheddar cheese, shredded
- 1/4 tsp garlic salt
- For dip:
- 1 1/2 tsp dijon mustard
- 1 tbsp mayonnaise

DIRECTIONS

1. Preheat your waffle maker.
2. Whisk eggs in a bowl.
3. Stir in ham, cheese, and garlic salt until combine.
4. Spray waffle maker with cooking spray.
5. Pour half of the batter in the hot waffle maker and cook for 3-4 minutes or until golden brown. Repeat with the remaining batter.
6. For dip: in a small bowl, mix mustard and mayonnaise.
7. Servings chaffle with dip.

NUTRITION: Calories 205 Fat 15.6 g Carbohydrates 3.4 g Sugar 0.9 g Protein 12.9 g Cholesterol 123 mg

36. Delicious Bagel Chaffle

Preparation Time: 15 minutes

Servings: 2

INGREDIENTS

- 1 egg, lightly beaten
- 1/4 tsp garlic powder
- 1/4 tsp onion powder
- 1 1/2 tsp bagel seasoning
- 3/4 cup mozzarella cheese, shredded
- 1/2 tsp baking powder, gluten-free
- 1 tbsp almond flour

DIRECTIONS

1. Preheat your waffle maker.
2. In a bowl, mix egg, bagel seasoning, baking powder, onion powder, garlic powder, and almond flour until well combined.
3. Add cheese and stir well.
4. Spray waffle maker with cooking spray.
5. Pour 1/2 of batter in the hot waffle maker and cook for 5 minutes or until golden brown. Repeat with the remaining batter.
6. Servings and enjoy.

NUTRITION: Calories 85 Fat 5.8 g Carbohydrates 2.4 g Sugar 0.5 g Protein 6.6 g Cholesterol 87 mg

37. <u>**Cheesy Garlic Bread Chaffle**</u>

Preparation Time: 15 minutes

Servings: 2

INGREDIENTS

- 1 egg, lightly beaten
- 1 tsp parsley, minced
- 2 tbsp parmesan cheese, grated
- 1 tbsp butter, melted
- 1/4 tsp garlic powder

- 1/4 tsp baking powder, gluten-free
- 1 tsp coconut flour
- 1/2 cup cheddar cheese, shredded

DIRECTIONS

1. Preheat your waffle maker.
2. In a bowl, whisk egg, garlic powder, baking powder, coconut flour, and cheddar cheese until well combined.
3. Spray waffle maker with cooking spray.
4. Pour half of the batter in the hot waffle maker and cook for 3 minutes or until set. Repeat with the remaining batter.
5. Brush chaffles with melted butter.
6. Place chaffles on baking tray and top with parmesan cheese and broil until cheese melted.
7. Garnish with parsley and servings.

NUTRITION: Calories 248 Fat 19.4 g Carbohydrates 5.4 g Sugar 1 g Protein 12.5 g Cholesterol 131 mg

38. Zucchini Basil Chaffle

Preparation Time: 15 minutes

Servings: 2

INGREDIENTS

- 1 egg, lightly beaten
- 1/4 cup fresh basil, chopped
- 1/4 cup mozzarella cheese, shredded
- 1/2 cup parmesan cheese, shredded
- 1 cup zucchini, grated and squeeze out all liquid
- 1/4 tsp pepper
- 3/4 tsp salt

DIRECTIONS

1. Preheat your waffle maker.
2. In a small bowl, beat the egg.
3. Add basil, mozzarella cheese, zucchini, pepper, and salt and stir well.
4. Spray waffle maker with cooking spray.
5. Sprinkle 2 tbsp of parmesan cheese to the bottom of waffle iron then spread 1/4 of the batter and top with 2 tbsp parmesan cheese and cook for 4-8 minutes or until set. Repeat with the remaining batter.
6. Servings and enjoy.

NUTRITION: Calories 218 Fat 13.9 g Carbohydrates 3.8 g Sugar 1.2 g Protein 19.7 g Cholesterol 113 mg

39.   Jicama chaffle

Preparation Time: 15 minutes

Servings: 2

INGREDIENTS

- 2 eggs, lightly beaten
- 1 cup cheddar cheese, shredded
- 1/4 tsp garlic powder
- 1/4 tsp onion powder
- 1 large jicama root, peel, shredded and squeeze out all liquid
- Pepper
- Salt

DIRECTIONS

1. Preheat your waffle maker.
2. Add shredded jicama in microwave-safe bowl and microwave for 5-8 minutes.
3. Add remaining ingredients to the bowl and stir to combine.

4. Spray waffle maker with cooking spray.
5. Pour half of the batter in the hot waffle maker and cook until golden brown or set. Repeat with the remaining batter.
6. Servings and enjoy.

NUTRITION: Calories 315 Fat 23.1 g Carbohydrates 7.1 g Sugar 2.3 g Protein 20.2 g Cholesterol 223 mg

40. <u>Tasty Broccoli Chaffle</u>

Preparation Time: 15 minutes

Servings: 3

INGREDIENTS

- 2 eggs, lightly beaten
- 1/3 cup parmesan cheese, grated
- 1 cup cheddar cheese, shredded
- 1 cup broccoli

DIRECTIONS

1. Preheat your waffle maker.
2. Add broccoli into the food processor and process until it looks like rice. Transfer broccoli into the mixing bowl.
3. Add remaining ingredients into the bowl and mix until well combined.
4. Spray waffle maker with cooking spray.
5. Pour 1/3 of batter in the hot waffle maker and cook for 4-5 minutes until golden brown. Repeat with the remaining batter.
6. Servings and enjoy.

NUTRITION: Calories 271 Fat 19.5 g Carbohydrates 2.7 g Sugar 1 g Protein 19.3 g Cholesterol 162 mg

41. Quick Carnivore Chaffle

Preparation Time: 10 minutes

Servings: 1

INGREDIENTS

- 1 egg, lightly beaten
- 1/3 cup cheddar cheese, shredded
- 1/2 cup ground pork rinds
- Pinch of salt

DIRECTIONS

1. Preheat your waffle maker.
2. In a bowl, whisk egg, pork rinds, cheese, and salt.
3. Spray waffle maker with cooking spray.
4. Pour batter in the hot waffle maker and cook for 5 minutes until golden brown.
5. Servings and enjoy.

NUTRITION: Calories 275 Fat 20.2 g Carbohydrates 0.8 g Sugar 0.5 g Protein 23.6 g Cholesterol 203 mg

42. Cinnamon chaffle

Preparation Time: 15 minutes

Servings: 2

INGREDIENTS

- 1 egg, lightly beaten
- 1/2 tsp vanilla
- 1/2 tsp cinnamon
- 1/2 cup mozzarella cheese, shredded

DIRECTIONS

1. Preheat your waffle maker.
2. In a small bowl, whisk egg, vanilla, cinnamon, and cheese until well combined.
3. Spray waffle maker with cooking spray.
4. Pour half batter in the hot waffle maker and cook until golden brown. Repeat with the remaining batter.
5. Servings and enjoy.

NUTRITION: Calories 56 Fat 3.5 g Carbohydrates 1 g Sugar 0.3 g Protein 4.8 g Cholesterol 86 mg

43.   Keto Breakfast Chaffle

Preparation Time: 3 minutes

Cooking Time: 6 minutes

Servings: 1

INGREDIENTS

- 2 tablespoons butter
- 1 egg
- 1/2 cup monterey jack cheese
- 1 tablespoon almond flour

DIRECTIONS

1. Preheat mini waffle maker until hot
2. Whisk egg in a bowl, add cheese, then mix well
3. Stir in the remaining ingredients (except toppings, if any).
4. Grease waffle maker and scoop 1/2 of the batter onto the waffle maker, spread across evenly
5. Cook until a bit browned and crispy, about 4 minutes.
6. Gently remove from waffle maker and let it cool
7. Repeat with remaining batter.

8. Melt butter in a pan. Add chaffles to the pan and cook for 2 minutes on each side
9. Remove from the pan and let it cool.
10. Servings and enjoy!

Nutrition: 257 Calories 1g Net Carbs 24g Fat 11g Protein

44. <u>Pumpkin chaffle</u>

Preparation Time: 5 minutes

Cooking Time: 5 minutes

Servings: 2

INGREDIENTS

- ½ cup mozzarella cheese, shredded
- 1 tablespoon coconut flour
- 1 egg, whisked
- 1 tablespoon stevia
- 2 tablespoons pumpkin puree
- 2 tablespoons cream cheese
- ½ teaspoon almond extract

DIRECTIONS

1. In a bowl, mix the mozzarella with the flour, egg and the other ingredients and whisk well.
2. Heat up the waffle iron over high heat, pour half of the batter, close the waffle maker, cook for 5 minutes and transfer to a plate.
3. Repeat with the other part of the batter and servings the chaffles warm.

NUTRITION: Calories 200, Fat 15, Fiber 1.2, Carbs 3.4, Protein 12.05

45.   Carrot Cake Chaffles

Preparation Time: 10 minutes

Cooking Time: 10 minutes

Servings: 4

INGREDIENTS

- 2 tablespoons cream cheese, soft
- ½ cup carrots, peeled and grated
- 2 tablespoons stevia
- 1 egg, whisked
- ½ teaspoon baking powder
- 3 tablespoons almond flour
- ½ cup heavy cream
- 1 tablespoon swerve

DIRECTIONS

1. In a bowl, mix the carrots with the cream cheese and the other ingredients except the heavy cream and swerve whisk.
2. Heat up the waffle iron, divide the batter into 4 parts and cook the chaffles.
3. In a bowl mix the heavy cream with the swerve and whisk.
4. Layer the chaffles and the cream and servings the cake cold.

NUTRITION: Calories 251, Fat 13, Fiber 2.3, Carbs 5, Protein 6

46.   Italian Garlic Chaffle

Preparation Time: 15 minutes

Servings: 2

INGREDIENTS

- 1 egg, lightly beaten
- 1/8 tsp italian seasoning
- 1/4 tsp garlic, minced
- 1/4 cup parmesan cheese, grated
- 1/2 cup mozzarella cheese, shredded

DIRECTIONS

1. Preheat your waffle maker.
2. In a small bowl, whisk egg, italian seasoning, garlic, parmesan cheese, and mozzarella cheese until well combined.
3. Spray waffle maker with cooking spray.
4. Pour half batter in the hot waffle maker and cook for 4-5 minutes or until golden brown. Repeat with the remaining batter.
5. Servings and enjoy.

NUTRITION: Calories 128 Fat 8 g Carbohydrates 0.6 g Sugar 0.2 g Protein 10.8 g Cholesterol 101 mg

47.   Tuna dill chaffle

Preparation Time: 15 minutes

Servings: 2

INGREDIENTS

- 1 egg, lightly beaten
- 1 dill pickle, sliced
- 1 tbsp mayonnaise
- 1/3 cup cheddar cheese, shredded
- 1 can tuna, drained

DIRECTIONS

1. Preheat your waffle maker.
2. Add all ingredients in mixing bowl and whisk until well combined.
3. Spray waffle maker with cooking spray.
4. Pour half batter in the hot waffle maker and cook for 5 minutes. Repeat with the remaining batter.
5. Servings and enjoy.

NUTRITION: Calories 305 Fat 18.1 g Carbohydrates 2.9 g Sugar 1.1 g Protein 31.3 g Cholesterol 131 mg

48. **Perfect Breakfast Chaffle**

Preparation Time: 15 minutes

Servings: 2

INGREDIENTS

- 1 egg, lightly beaten
- 1/2 tsp baking powder, gluten-free
- 1 tbsp almond flour
- 1/4 cup mozzarella cheese, shredded
- 1/4 cup cheddar cheese, shredded
- 1/4 tsp onion powder
- 1/4 tsp garlic powder
- 1/4 tsp cinnamon
- Pepper
- Salt

DIRECTIONS

1. Preheat your waffle maker.
2. Add all ingredients into the mixing bowl and mix well.
3. Spray waffle maker with cooking spray.
4. Pour half batter in the hot waffle maker and cook until golden brown. Repeat with the remaining batter.
5. Servings and enjoy.

NUTRITION: Calories 123 Fat 9.3 g Carbohydrates 2.6 g Sugar 0.6 g Protein 8.2 g Cholesterol 99 mg

49. Coconut Scallion Chaffle

Preparation Time: 15 minutes

Servings: 2

INGREDIENTS

- 1 egg, lightly beaten
- 1 ½ tsp coconut flour
- 2 tbsp scallions, sliced
- 1 cup cheddar cheese, shredded
- 1 cup mozzarella cheese, shredded
- Pepper
- Salt

DIRECTIONS

1. Preheat your waffle maker.
2. Add all ingredients in a bowl and mix well.
3. Spray waffle maker with cooking spray.
4. Pour half batter in the hot waffle maker and cook until golden brown. Repeat with the remaining batter.
5. Servings and enjoy.

NUTRITION: Calories 346 Fat 24.9 g Carbohydrates 7.9 g Sugar 1.4 g Protein 22.5 g Cholesterol 149 mg

50. Jalapeno Ham Chaffle

Preparation Time: 20 minutes

Servings: 4

INGREDIENTS

- 2 eggs, lightly beaten
- 2 tsp coconut flour
- 1 tbsp green onion, chopped
- 2 oz ham, chopped
- 1/2 jalapeno pepper, grated
- 2 oz cheddar cheese, shredded

DIRECTIONS

1. Preheat your waffle maker.
2. Add all ingredients into the mixing bowl and mix until well combined.
3. Spray waffle maker with cooking spray.
4. Pour 1/4 of the batter in the hot waffle maker and cook for 3-4 minutes or until golden brown. Repeat with the remaining batter.
5. Servings and enjoy.

NUTRITION: Calories 143 Fat 9.1 g Carbohydrates 5.1 g Sugar 0.8 g Protein 9.7 g Cholesterol 105 mg

51. Tasty Jalapeno Chaffle

Preparation Time: 10 minutes

Servings: 1

INGREDIENTS

- 1 egg, lightly beaten
- 1 tbsp olive oil
- 1 tbsp jalapeno, chopped
- 1 tbsp almond flour
- 1/2 cup cheddar cheese, shredded

DIRECTIONS

1. Preheat your waffle maker.
2. Add all ingredients into the bowl and whisk until well combined.
3. Spray waffle maker with cooking spray.
4. Pour batter in the hot waffle maker and cook until golden brown.
5. Servings and enjoy.

NUTRITION: Calories 465 Fat 43.9 g Carbohydrates 4.2 g Sugar 0.8 g Protein 21.1 g Cholesterol 234 mg

52. Crispy chaffle

Preparation Time: 15 minutes

Servings: 4

INGREDIENTS

- 2 eggs, lightly beaten
- 1 cup cheddar cheese, shredded
- 1/4 tsp baking powder, gluten-free
- 1/4 cup almond flour

DIRECTIONS

1. Preheat your waffle maker and spray with cooking spray.
2. In a bowl, whisk eggs, baking powder, and almond flour.
3. Add cheese and stir to combine.
4. Pour 1/4 of the batter in the hot waffle maker and cook until golden brown. Repeat with the remaining batter.
5. Servings and enjoy.

NUTRITION: Calories 186 Fat 15.1 g Carbohydrates 2.2 g Sugar 0.6 g Protein 11.3 g Cholesterol 112 mg

53.   Crispy Cheddar Cheese Chaffle

Preparation Time: 13 minutes

Servings: 1

INGREDIENTS

- 1 egg, lightly beaten
- 2 oz cheddar cheese, thinly sliced

DIRECTIONS

1. Preheat your waffle maker and spray with cooking spray.
2. Arrange half cheese slices on hot waffle maker then pour the egg on top.
3. Now place remaining cheese slices on top and cook for 6-8 minutes.
4. Servings and enjoy.

NUTRITION: Calories 291 Fat 23.2 g Carbohydrates 1.1 g Sugar 0.6 g Protein 19.7 g Cholesterol 223 mg

CAKE CHAFFLES

54.   Keto Birthday Cake Chaffle Recipe with Sprinkles

Preparation Time: 10 minutes

Cooking Time: 7 minutes

Servings: 4

INGREDIENTS

Ingredients for chaffle cake:

- 2 eggs
- 1/4 almond flour
- 1 cup coconut powder
- 1 cup melted butter
- 2 tablespoons cream cheese
- 1 teaspoon cake butter extract
- 1 tsp vanilla extract
- 2 tsp baking powder
- 2 teaspoons confectionery sweetener or monk fruit
- 1/4 teaspoon xanthan powder whipped cream

Vanilla frosting ingredients

- 1/2 cup heavy whipped cream
- 2 tablespoons sweetener or monk fruit
- 1/2 teaspoon vanilla extract

PREPARATION

1. The mini waffle maker is preheated.
2. Add all the ingredients of the chaffle cake in a medium-sized blender and blend it to the top until it is smooth and creamy. Allow only a minute to sit with the

batter. It may seem a little watery, but it's going to work well.

3. Add 2 to 3 tablespoons of batter to your waffle maker and cook until golden brown for about 2 to 3 minutes.
4. Start to frost the whipped vanilla cream in a separate bowl.
5. Add all the ingredients and mix with a hand mixer until thick and soft peaks are formed by the whipping cream.
6. Until frosting your cake, allow the keto birthday cake chaffles to cool completely. If you frost it too soon, the frosting will be melted.
7. Enjoy! Enjoy!

NUTRITION: Calories 141, total Fat 10.2g, cholesterol 111mg, sodium 55.7mg, total carbohydrate 4.7g, dietary Fiber 0.4g, sugars 0.8g, Protein 4.7g, vitamin a 96.6µg, vitamin c 0mg

55. Keto Chocolate Waffle Cake

Preparation Time: 5 minutes

Cooking Time: 5 minutes

Servings: 3

INGREDIENTS

1. 2 tbs cocoa
2. 2 tbs monkfruit confectioner's
3. 1 egg
4. 1/4 teaspoon baking powder
5. 1 tbs heavy whipped cream

Frosted ingredients

6. 2 tbs monkfruit confectioners
7. 2 tbs cream cheese softens, room temperature
8. 1/4 teaspoon transparent vanilla

PREPARATION

1. Whip the egg in a small bowl.
2. Add the rest of the ingredients and mix well until smooth and creamy.
3. Pour half of the batter into a mini waffle maker and cook until fully cooked for 2 1/2 to 3 minutes.
4. Add the sweetener, cream cheese, and vanilla in a separate small bowl. Mix the frosting until all is well embedded.
5. Spread the frosting on the cake after it has cooled down to room temperature.

NUTRITION: Calories 120, total Fat 10.5g, cholesterol 87.2mg, sodium 87.3mg, total carbohydrate 9.2g, dietary Fiber 1.4g, sugars 1.1g, Protein 4.1g, vitamin a 106.8µg, vitamin c 0mg

56.   Keto Vanilla Twinkie Copycat Chaffle

Preparation Time: 5 minutes

Cooking Time: 4 minutes

Servings: 4

INGREDIENTS

- 2 tablespoons of butter (cooled)
- 2 oz cream cheese softened
- Two large egg room temperature
- 1 teaspoon of vanilla essence
- Optional 1/2 teaspoon vanilla cupcake extract
- 1/4 cup lacanto confectionery
- Pinch of salt
- 1/4 cup almond flour
- 2 tablespoons coconut powder

1 teaspoon baking powder

DIRECTIONS

1. Preheat corndog maker.
2. Melt the butter and let cool for 1 minute.
3. Whisk the butter until the eggs are creamy.
4. Add vanilla, extract, sweetener and salt and mix well.
5. Add almond flour, coconut flour, baking powder.
6. Mix until well incorporated.
7. Add ~ 2 tbs batter to each well and spread evenly.
8. Close and lock the lid and cook for 4 minutes.
9. Remove and cool the rack.

NUTRITION: Calories 152, total Fat 9g, cholesterol 100.7mg, sodium 727.7mg, total carbohydrate 6.5g, dietary Fiber 1.6g, sugars 2.4g, Protein 6.1g, vitamin a 120.2µg, vitamin c 0mg

57. Carrot Chaffle Cake

Preparation Time: 5 minutes

Cooking Time: 5 minutes

Servings: 6

INGREDIENTS

- 1/2 cup chopped carrot
- 1 egg
- 2 t butter melted
- 2 t heavy whipped cream
- 3/4 cup almond flour
- 1 walnut chopped
- 2 t powder sweetener
- 2 tsp cinnamon
- 1 tsp pumpkin spice
- 1 tsp baking powder
- Cream cheese frosting
- 4 oz cream cheese softened
- 1/4 cup powdered sweetener

- 1 teaspoon of vanilla essence
- 1-2 t heavy whipped cream according to your preferred consistency

DIRECTIONS

1. Mix dry ingredients such as almond flour, cinnamon, pumpkin spices, baking powder, powdered sweeteners, and walnut pieces.
2. Add the grated carrots, eggs, melted butter and cream.
3. Add a 3t batter to a preheated mini waffle maker. Cook for 2 1 / 2-3 minutes.
4. Mix the frosted ingredients with a hand mixer with a whisk until well mixed
5. Stack waffles and add a frost between each layer!

Note: (serving) 2.4 non-freezing net carbohydrates, 3.7 net Carbs with icing, 1/4 of the cake are 5.5 net carbs!

58.   Easy Soft Cinnamon Rolls Chaffle Cake

Preparation Time: 5 minutes

Cooking Time: 12 minutes

Servings: 3

INGREDIENTS

- 1 egg
- 1/2 cup mozzarella cheese
- 1/2 tsp vanilla
- 1/2 tsp cinnamon
- 1 tbs monk fruit confectioners blend

DIRECTIONS

1. Put the eggs in a small bowl.
2. Add the remaining ingredients.

3. Spray to the waffle maker with a non-stick cooking spray.
4. Make two chaffles.
5. Separate the mixture.
6. Cook half of the mixture for about 4 minutes or until golden.
1. Notes added glaze: 1 tb of cream cheese melted in a microwave for 15 seconds, and 1 tb of monk fruit confectioners mix. Mix it and spread it over the moist fabric.
2. Additional frosting: 1 tb cream cheese (high temp), 1 tb room temp butter (low temp) and 1 tb mmonk fruit confectioners' mix. Mix all the ingredients together and spread to the top of the cloth.
3. Top with optional frosting, glaze, nuts, sugar-free syrup, whipped cream or simply dust with monk fruit sweets.

NUTRITION: Calories 106, total Fat 6.6g, cholesterol 107mg, sodium 182.3mg, total carbohydrate 4.6g, dietary Fiber 0.3g, sugars 2.7g, Protein 8.2g, vitamin a 94.7μg, vitamin c 0mg

59. <u>Banana Pudding Chaffle Cake</u>

Preparation Time: 5 minutes

Cooking Time: 5 minutes

Servings: 2

INGREDIENTS

- 1 large egg yolk
- 1/2 cup fresh cream
- 3 t powder sweetener
- 1 / 4-1 / 2 teaspoon xanthan gum
- 1/2 teaspoon banana extract
- Banana chaffle ingredients
- 1 oz softened cream cheese
- 1/4 cup mozzarella cheese shredded
- 1 egg

- 1 teaspoon banana extract
- 2 t sweetener
- 1 tsp baking powder
- 4 t almond flour

PREPARATIONS

1. Mix heavy cream, powdered sweetener and egg yolk in a small pot. Whisk constantly until the sweetener has dissolved and the mixture is thick.
2. Cook for 1 minute. Add xanthan gum and whisk.
3. Remove from heat, add a pinch of salt and banana extract and stir well.
4. Transfer to a glass dish and cover the pudding with plastic wrap. Refrigerate.
5. Mix all ingredients together. Cook in a preheated mini waffle maker.

Note: Make three chaffles. 3.3 net Carbs / serving. Recipe 9.8 net Carbs

60.   Keto Peanut Butter Chaffle Cake

Preparation Time: 5 minutes

Cooking Time: 5 minutes

Servings: 2

INGREDIENTS

Ingredients for peanut butter chaffle:

- 2 tbs sugar free peanut butter powder
- 2 tbs monkfruit confectioner 's
- 1 egg
- 1/4 teaspoon baking powder
- 1 tbs heavy whipped cream
- 1/4 teaspoon peanut butter extract

- Peanut butter frosting ingredients
- 2 tbs monkfruit confectioners
- 1 tbs butter softens, room temperature
- 1 tbs unsweetened natural peanut butter or peanut butter powder
- 2 tbs cream cheese softens, room temperature
- 1/4 tsp vanilla

DIRECTIONS

1. Serve the eggs in a small bowl.
2. Add the remaining ingredients and mix well until the dough is smooth and creamy.
3. If you don't have peanut butter extract, you can skip it. It adds absolutely wonderful, more powerful peanut butter flavor and is worth investing in this extract.
4. Pour half of the butter into a mini waffle maker and cook for 2-3 minutes until it is completely cooked.
5. In another small bowl, add sweetener, cream cheese, sugar-free natural peanut butter and vanilla. Mix frosting until everything is well incorporated.
6. When the waffle cake has completely cooled to room temperature, spread the frosting.
7. Or you can even pipe the frost!
8. Or you can heat the frosting and add 1/2 teaspoon of water to make the peanut butter aze pill and drizzle over the peanut butter chaffle! I like it anyway!

NUTRITION: Calories 92, total Fat 7g, cholesterol 97.1mg, sodium 64.3mg, total carbohydrate 3.6g, dietary Fiber 0.6g, sugars 1.8g, Protein 5.5g, vitamin a 52.1µg, vitamin c 0mg

61.   Keto Italian Cream Chaffle Cake

Preparation Time: 5 minutes

Cooking Time: 3 minutes

Servings: 1

INGREDIENTS

For sweet chaffle:

1. 4 oz cream cheese softens, room temperature
2. 4 eggs
3. 1 tablespoon butter
4. 1 teaspoon of vanilla essence
5. 1/2 teaspoon of cinnamon
6. 1 tbsp monk fruit sweetener or favorite keto approved sweetener
7. 4 tablespoons coconut powder
8. 1 tablespoon almond flour
9. 1 1/2 cup baking powder
10. 1 tablespoon coconut
11. 1 walnut chopped
12. Italian cream frosting ingredients
13. 2 oz. Cream cheese softens, room temperature
14. 2 cups of butter room temp
15. 2 tbs monk fruit sweetener or favorite keto approved sweetener
16. 1/2 teaspoon vanilla

DIRECTIONS

1. In a medium blender, add cream cheese, eggs, melted butter, vanilla, sweeteners, coconut flour, almond flour, and baking powder. Optional: add shredded coconut and walnut to the mixture or save for matting. Both methods are great!
2. Mix the ingredients high until smooth and creamy.
3. Preheat mini waffle maker.
4. Add ingredients to the preheated waffle maker.
5. Cook for about 2-3 minutes until the waffle is complete.
6. Remove chaffle and let cool.
7. In a separate bowl, add all the ingredients together and start frosting. Stir until smooth and creamy.
8. When the chaffle has cooled completely, frost the cake.

Note: Create 8 mini chaffles or 3-4 large chaffles.

NUTRITION: Calories 127, total Fat 9.7g, cholesterol 102.9mg, sodium 107.3mg, total carbohydrate 5.5g, dietary Fiber 1.3g, sugars 1.5g, Protein 5.3g, vitamin a 99μg, vitamin c 0.1mg

62.   Keto Boston Cream Pie Chaffle Cake

PREPARATION Time: 10 minutes

Cooking Time: 5 minutes

Servings: 4

INGREDIENTS

Ingredients for chaffle cake:

- 2 eggs
- 1/4 cup almond flour
- Coconut flower 1 teaspoon
- 2 tablespoons of melted butter
- 2 tablespoons of cream cheese
- 20 drops of boston cream extract
- 1/2 teaspoon of vanilla essence
- 1/2 teaspoon baking powder
- 2 tablespoons sweetener or monk fruit
- 1/4 teaspoon xanthan powder

Custard ingredients

- 1/2 cup fresh cream
- 1/2 teaspoon of vanilla essence
- 1/2 tbs swerve confectioner's sweetener
- 2 yolks
- 1/8 teaspoon xanthan gum

Ingredients for ganache:

- 2 tbs heavy whipped cream

- 2 tbs unsweetened baking chocolate bar chopped
- 1 tbs swerve confectioners sweetener

INGREDIENTS

1. Preheat the mini waffle iron to render the cake chops first.

2. In a mixer, mix all the ingredients of the cake and blend until smooth and fluffy. It's only supposed to take a few minutes.

3. Heat the heavy whipping cream to a boil on the stovetop. While it's dry, whisk the egg yolks together in a small separate dish.

4. Once the cream is boiling, add half of it to the egg yolks. Make sure you're whisking it together while you're slowly pouring it into the mixture.

5. Add the egg and milk mixture to the rest of the cream in the stovetop pan and stir vigorously for another 2-3 minutes.

6. Take the custard off the heat and whisk in your vanilla and xanthan gum. Then set aside to cool and thicken.

7. Place the ganache ingredients in a small bowl. Microwave for about 20 seconds, stir. Repeat, if necessary. Careful not to overheat and roast the ganache. Just do it 20 seconds at a time until it's completely melted.

8. Assemble and enjoy your boston cream pie chaffle cake!

63. <u>Keto Birthday Cake Chaffle</u>

Preparation Time: 10 minutes

Cooking Time: 5 minutes

Servings: 4

INGREDIENTS

Ingredients for chaffle cake:

- 2 eggs
- 1/4 cup almond flour
- Coconut flower 1 teaspoon
- 2 tablespoons of melted butter
- 2 tablespoons of cream cheese
- 1 teaspoon cake batter extract
- 1/2 teaspoon of vanilla essence
- 1/2 teaspoon baking powder
- 2 tablespoons sweetener or monk fruit
- 1/4 teaspoon xanthan powder
- Whipped cream vanilla frosting ingredients
- 1/2 cup fresh cream
- 2 tablespoons 2 tablespoons sweets sweetener or monk fruit
- 1/2 teaspoon of vanilla essence

DIRECTIONS

1. Preheat mini waffle maker.
2. In a medium sized blender, add all the ingredients of the chaffle cake and blend high until smooth and creamy. Let the dough sit for only one minute. It may look a bit watery, but it works.
3. Add 2-3 tablespoons of dough to the waffle maker and cook for about 2-3 minutes until golden.
4. In another bowl, start making the whipped cream vanilla frosting.
5. Add all ingredients and mix with hand mixer until whipped cream thickens and soft peaks form.
6. Let the keto birthday cake chaffle cool completely before frosting the cake. If the frost is too early, the frost will melt.
7. Pleasant!

NUTRITION: Calories 141, total Fat 10.2g, cholesterol 111mg, sodium 55.7mg, total carbohydrate 4.7g, dietary Fiber 0.4g, sugars 0.8g, Protein 4.7g, vitamin a 96.6µg, vitamin c 0mg

64.   Keto Strawberry Shortcake Chaffle

Preparation Time: 2 minutes

Cooking Time: 4 minutes

Servings: 2

INGREDIENTS

- 1 egg
- 1 tablespoon heavy whipped cream
- 1 tsp coconut flour
- 2 tablespoons of lacanto golden sweetener (use off wine)
- 1/2 teaspoon cake batter extract
- 1/4 teaspoon baking powder

DIRECTIONS

1. Preheat the maker of mini waffles.
2. Combine all the ingredients of the chaffle in a small bowl.
3. Pour half of the mixture of the chaffle into the waffle iron center. Allow 3-5 minutes to cook. If the chaffle rises, lift the lid slightly for a couple of seconds until it begins to go back down and restore the lid as it finishes.
4. Carefully remove the second chaffle and repeat it. Let the chaffles sit for a couple of minutes to crisp up.
5. Add your desired and enjoyed amount of whipped cream and strawberries!
6. Notes: recipe is perfect in a standard waffle maker for either two mini chaffles or one chaffle.
7. The calculated macros on the bottom are before the amount of strawberries and whipped cream you want.

NUTRITION: Calories 268, total Fat 11.8g, cholesterol 121mg, sodium 221.8mg, Total carbohydrate 5.1g, dietary Fiber 1.7g, sugars 1.2g, Protein 10g, vitamin a 133.5µg, vitamin c 7.3mg

65.   Sloppy Joe Chaffle

Preparation Time: 10 minutes

Cooking Time: 5 minutes

Servings: 4

INGREDIENTS

- Sloppy jaw ingredients
- 1 lb ground beef
- 1 tsp onion powder
- 1 teaspoon of garlic
- 3 tbsp tomato paste
- 1/2 teaspoon
- 1/4 teaspoon pepper
- Chili powder 1 tbs
- 1 teaspoon of cocoa powder this is optional but highly recommended! It enhances the flavor!
- Usually 1/2 cup bone soup beef flavor
- 1 teaspoon coconut amino or soy sauce as you like
- 1 teaspoon mustard powder
- 1 teaspoon of brown or screen golden
- 1/2 teaspoon paprika

Ingredients for corn bread chaffle

- Make two chaffles
- 1 egg
- 1/2 cup cheddar cheese
- 5-slice jalapeno, very small diced (pickled or fresh)
- 1 tsp frank red hot sauce

- 1/4 teaspoon corn extract is optional, but tastes like real cornbread!
- Pinch salt

DIRECTIONS

- First, cook the minced meat with salt and pepper.
- Add all remaining ingredients.
- Cook the mixture while making the chaffle.
- Preheating waffle maker.
- Put the eggs in a small bowl.
- Add the remaining ingredients.
- Spray to the waffle maker with a non-stick cooking spray.
- Divide the mixture in half.
- Simmer half of the mixture for about 4 minutes or until golden.
- For a chaffled crispy rind, add 1 teaspoon cheese to the waffle maker for 30 seconds before adding the mixture.
- Pour the warm stubby joe mix into the hot chaffle and finish! Dinner is ready! !

Note: You can also add diced jalapenos (fresh or pickled) to this basic chaffle recipe to make a jalapeno cornbread chaffle recipe!

NUTRITION: Calories156, total Fat 3.9g, cholesterol 67.8mg, sodium 392.6mg, total carbohydrate 3.9g, dietary Fiber 1.2g, sugars 1.6g, Protein 25.8g, vitamin a 33.1µg, vitamin c 3.1mg,

66.   Bacon Egg & Cheese Chaffle

Preparation Time: 3 minutes

Cooking Time: 7 minutes

Servings: 2

INGREDIENTS

1. 3/4 of a chopped chess cup (i used a blend of sharp cheddar and mozzarella cheese) 2 eggs (scrambled) 3 slices of thin bacon. Waffle iron)
2. A pinch of salt
3. 1/4 teaspoon pepper

DIRECTIONS

1. Directions cut small pieces of bacon. Scramble the egg in a medium-sized bowl and mix salt and pepper in the cheese, then add the pieces of bacon and mix them all together.
2. Preheat your waffle iron when it is open at the proper cooking temperature and pour the mixture into the center of the iron to ensure that it is distributed evenly
3. Close your waffle iron and set the timer for 4 minutes and do not open too quickly. No matter how good it begins to smell, let it cook. A good rule to follow is that if the waffle machine stops steaming, the chaffle will be done.
4. When the time is up, gently open the waffle iron and make sure not all of it sticks to the top. If so, use a teflon or other non-metallic spatula to pry the chaffle softly away from the top and then gently pull the chaffle from the bottom and onto the plate after you have fully opened the unit.

NUTRITION: Calories 490, Calories from Fat 141, Fat 15.7g, sodium 209mg, potassium 128mg, carbohydrates 9.9g Fiber 2.9g, sugar 0.9g, Protein 11.5g, vitamin a 345iu, calcium 175mg, iron 1.8mg

67. Crunchy Keto Cinnamon Chaffle

Preparation Time: 5 minutes

Cooking Time: 10 minutes

Servings: 2

INGREDIENTS

- 1 tablespoon almond flour
- 1 egg
- 1 teaspoon of vanilla
- Cinnamon 1 shake
- 1 teaspoon baking powder
- 1 cup mozzarella cheese

INGREDIENTS

1. Mix the egg and vanilla extract in a bowl.
2. Mix powder, almond flour and cinnamon with baking.
3. Finally, add the cheese in the mozzarella and coat with the mixture evenly.
4. Spray oil on your waffle maker and let it heat up to its maximum setting.
5. Cook the waffle, test it every 5 minutes until it becomes golden and crunchy. A tip: make sure you put half of the batter in it. It can overflow the waffle maker, rendering it a sloppy operation. I suggest you put down a silpat mat to make it easy to clean.
6. With butter and your favorite low-carb syrup, take it out carefully.

NUTRITION: Calories 450, Calories from Fat 141, Fat 15.7g, sodium 209mg, potassium 128mg, carbohydrates 9.9g, Fiber 2.9g, sugar 0.9g, Protein 11.5g, vitamin a 345iu, calcium 175mg, iron 1.8mg

68.   Crispy Burger Bun Chaffle

Preparation Time: 5 minutes

Cooking Time: 14 minutes

Servings: 1

INGREDIENTS

- 1 egg
- 1/2 cup mozzarella cheese shredded
- 1/4 teaspoon baking powder
- 1/4 teaspoon glucomannan powder
- 1/4 teaspoon allulose or other sweetener
- 1/4 teaspoon caraway seed or other seasoning

DIRECTIONS

1. In a pot, add all the ingredients and blend together with a fork.
2. Spoon part of the mixture into the waffle maker, depending on whether you want them soft or crispy, cook for 5 to 7 minutes.
3. Prepare as you usually do your burger. Usually i cook a bacon strip in a cast iron pan and then fry a burger over medium low heat with salt and pepper in the bacon fat. I add the cheese a couple of minutes after frying, pour in a 1/4 cup of water and place a metal bowl over the burger to steam the cheese. I like my burgers with lettuce, tomato, onion, a bit of ranch dressing, salt, and pepper. But, that's me. You're doing it.
4. Pop it in the toaster oven when the first chaffle comes out to keep it warm while the second chaffle is being made, again for 5 to 7 minutes.

NUTRITION: Calories 258, Calories from Fat 141, Fat 15.7g, sodium 209mg, potassium 128mg, carbohydrates 9.9g, Fiber 2.9g, sugar 0.9g, Protein 11.5g, vitamin a 345iu, calcium 175mg, iron 1.8mg

69. Vegan Keto Chaffle Waffle

Preparation Time: 5 minutes

Cooking Time: 5 minutes

Servings: 2

INGREDIENTS

- 1 tablespoon flax seed
- 2 glasses of water
- ¼ cup low carb vegan cheese
- 22 tablespoons coconut powder
- 1 1 tbsp low carb vegan cream cheese
- A pinch of salt

DIRECTIONS

1. Preheat the waffle maker to medium high heat.
2. In a small bowl, mix flax seed meal and water. Leave for 5 minutes until thick and sticky.
3. Make flax eggs
4. Whisk all vegan chaffle ingredients together.
5. Meat vegan keto waffle
6. Pour vegan waffle dough into the center of the waffle iron. Close the waffle maker and cook for 3-5 minutes or until the waffles are golden and firm. If using a mini waffle maker, pour only half the dough.
7. Pour the waffle mixture into the waffle maker
8. Remove the vegan chaffle from the waffle maker and serve.
9. You can eat vegan keto chaffles

NUTRITION: Calories 168, total Fat 11.8g, cholesterol 121mg, sodium 221.8mg, total carbohydrate 5.1g, dietary Fiber 1.7g, sugars 1.2g, Protein 10g, vitamin a 133.5µg, vitamin c 7.3mg

70. Pumpkin Cake Chaffle With Cream Cheese Frosting

Preparation Time: 15 minutes

Cooking Time: 28 minutes

Servings: 4

INGREDIENTS

For the pumpkin chaffles:

- 2 eggs, beaten
- ½ tsp pumpkin pie spice
- 1 cup finely grated mozzarella cheese
- 1 tbsp pumpkin puree
- For the cream cheese frosting:
- 2 tbsp cream cheese, softened
- 2 tbsp swerve confectioner's sugar
- ½ tsp vanilla extract

DIRECTIONS
For the chaffles:

1. Preheat the waffle iron.
2. In a medium bowl, mix the egg, pumpkin pie spice, mozzarella cheese, and pumpkin puree.
3. Open the iron and add a quarter of the mixture. Close and cook until crispy, 7 minutes.
4. Transfer the chaffle to a plate and make 3 more chaffles with the remaining batter.
5. For the cream cheese frosting:
6. Add the cream cheese, swerve sugar, and vanilla to a medium bowl and whisk using an electric mixer until smooth and fluffy.
7. Layer the chaffles one on another but with some frosting spread between the layers. Top with the bit of frosting.
8. Slice and serve.

NUTRITION: Calories 106 Fats 5.17g Carbs 1.9gnet Carbs 1.2g Protein 12.82g

71.   Birthday Cake Chaffles

Preparation Time: 15 minutes

Cooking Time: 28 minutes

Servings: 4

INGREDIENTS

For the chaffles:

- 2 eggs, beaten
- 1 cup finely grated swiss cheese
- For the frosting and topping:
- ½ cup heavy cream
- 2 tbsp sugar-free maple syrup
- ½ tsp vanilla extract
- 3 tbsp funfetti

DIRECTIONS
For the chaffles:

1. Preheat the waffle iron.
2. In a medium bowl, mix the egg and swiss cheese.
3. Open the iron and add a quarter of the mixture. Close and cook until crispy, 7 minutes.
4. Transfer the chaffle to a plate and make 3 more chaffles with the remaining batter.

For the frosting and topping:

5. Add the heavy cream, maple syrup, and vanilla extract in a medium bowl and whisk using an electric mixer until smooth and fluffy.
6. Layer the chaffles one on another but with some frosting spread between the layers.
7. top with the remaining bit of frosting and garnish with the funfetti.

NUTRITION: Calories 210 Fats 16.82g Carbs 2.42g Net Carbs 2.42g Protein 11.96g

72. S'mores Chaffles

Preparation Time: 15 minutes

Cooking Time: 28 minutes

Servings: 4

INGREDIENTS

- 2 eggs, beaten
- 1 cup finely grated gruyere cheese
- ½ tsp vanilla extract
- 2 tbsp swerve brown sugar
- A pinch of salt
- ¼ cup unsweetened chocolate chips, melted
- 2 tbsp low carb marshmallow fluff

DIRECTIONS

1. Preheat the waffle iron.
2. In a medium bowl, mix the eggs, gruyere cheese, vanilla, swerve sugar, and salt.
3. Open the iron and add a quarter of the mixture. Close and cook until crispy, 7 minutes.
4. Transfer the chaffle to a plate and make 3 more chaffles with the remaining batter.
5. Spread half of the chocolate on two chaffles, add the marshmallow fluff and cover with the other chaffles.
6. Swirl the remaining chocolate, slice in half and serve.

NUTRITION: Calories 203Fats 15.49g Carbs 0.95gNet Carbs 0.95g Protein 14.32g

73. Chocolate Cake Chaffles With Cream Cheese Frosting

Preparation Time: 10 minutes

Cooking Time: 28 minutes

Servings: 4

INGREDIENTS

For the chaffles:

- 2 eggs, beaten
- 1 cup finely grated gouda cheese
- 2 tsp unsweetened cocoa powder
- ¼ tsp sugar-free maple syrup
- 1 tbsp cream cheese, softened
- For the frosting:
- 3 tbsp cream cheese, softened
- ¼ tsp vanilla extract
- 2 tbsp sugar-free maple syrup

DIRECTIONS
For the chaffles:

1. Preheat the waffle iron.
2. In a medium bowl, mix all the ingredients for the chaffles.
3. Open the iron and add a quarter of the mixture. Close and cook until crispy, 7 minutes.
4. Transfer the chaffle to a plate and make 3 more chaffles with the remaining batter.
5. For the frosting:
6. In a medium bowl, beat the cream cheese, vanilla extract, and maple syrup with a hand mixer until smooth.
7. Assemble the chaffles with the frosting to make the cake making sure to top the last layer with some frosting.
8. Slice and serve.

NUTRITION: Calories 78 Fats 6.5g Carbs 1.24g Net Carbs 0.94g Protein 3.99g

74.   Lemon Cake Chaffle With Lemon Frosting

Preparation Time: 10 minutes

Cooking Time: 28 minutes

Servings: 4

INGREDIENTS

For the chaffles:

- 2 eggs, beaten
- ½ cup finely grated swiss cheese
- 2 oz cream cheese, softened
- ½ tsp lemon extract
- 20 drops cake batter extract
- For the frosting:
- ½ cup heavy cream
- 1 tbsp sugar-free maple syrup
- ¼ tsp lemon extract

DIRECTIONS
For the chaffles:

1. Preheat the waffle iron.
2. In a medium bowl, mix all the ingredients for the chaffles.
3. Open the iron and add a quarter of the mixture. Close and cook until crispy, 7 minutes.
4. Transfer the chaffle to a plate and make 3 more chaffles with the remaining batter.

For the frosting:

5. In a medium bowl, using a hand mixer, beat the heavy cream, maple syrup, and lemon extract until fluffy.
6. Assemble the chaffles with the frosting to make the cake.
7. Slice and serve.

NUTRITION: Calories 176Fats 15.18gCarbs 2.88gNet Carbs 2.88gProtein 7.63g

75.   Red Velvet Chaffle Cake

Preparation Time: 15 minutes

Cooking Time: 28 minutes

Servings: 4

INGREDIENTS

For the chaffles:

- 2 eggs, beaten
- ½ cup finely grated parmesan cheese
- 2 oz cream cheese, softened
- 2 drops red food coloring
- 1 tsp vanilla extract

For the frosting:

- 3 tbsp cream cheese, softened
- 1 tbsp sugar-free maple syrup
- ¼ tsp vanilla extract

DIRECTIONS
For the chaffles:

1. Preheat the waffle iron.
2. In a medium bowl, mix all the ingredients for the chaffles.
3. Open the iron and add a quarter of the mixture. Close and cook until crispy, 7 minutes.
4. Transfer the chaffle to a plate and make 3 more chaffles with the remaining batter.

For the frosting:

5. In a medium bowl, using a hand mixer, whisk the cream cheese, maple syrup, and vanilla extract until smooth.
6. Assemble the chaffles with the frosting to make the cake.
7. Slice and serve.

NUTRITION: Calories 147Fats 9.86gCarbs 5.22gNet Carbs 5.22gProtein 8.57g

76. Almond Butter Chaffle Cake with Chocolate Butter Frosting

Preparation Time: 20 minutes

Cooking Time: 28 minutes

Servings: 4

INGREDIENTS

For the chaffles:

- 1 egg, beaten
- ⅓ cup finely grated mozzarella cheese
- 1 tbsp almond flour
- 2 tbsp almond butter
- 1 tbsp swerve confectioner's sugar
- ½ tsp vanilla extract

For the chocolate butter frosting:

- 1½ cups butter, room temperature
- 1 cup unsweetened cocoa powder
- ½ cup almond milk
- 5 cups swerve confectioner's sugar
- 2 tsp vanilla extract

DIRECTIONS
For the chaffles:

1. Preheat the waffle iron.
2. In a medium bowl, mix the egg, mozzarella cheese, almond flour, almond butter, swerve confectioner's sugar, and vanilla extract.
3. Open the iron and add a quarter of the mixture. Close and cook until crispy, 7 minutes.
4. Transfer the chaffle to a plate and make 3 more chaffles with the remaining batter.

For the frosting:

5. In a medium bowl, cream the butter and cocoa powder until smooth.
6. Gradually, whisk in the almond milk and swerve confectioner's sugar until smooth.
7. Add the vanilla extract and mix well.
8. Assemble the chaffles with the frosting to make the cake.
9. Slice and serve.

NUTRITION: Calories 838Fats 85.35gCarbs 8.73gNet Carbs 2.03gProtein 13.59g

77. Cinnamon Chaffles With Custard Filling

Preparation Time: 25 minutes

Cooking Time: 28 minutes

Servings: 4

INGREDIENTS

For the custard filling:

- 4 egg yolks, beaten
- 1 tbsp erythritol
- ¼ tsp xanthan gum
- 1 cup heavy cream
- 1 tbsp vanilla extract

For the chaffles:

- 2 eggs, beaten
- 2 tbsp cream cheese, softened
- 1 cup finely grated monterey jack cheese
- 1 tsp vanilla extract
- 1 tbsp heavy cream
- 1 tbsp coconut flour

- ½ tsp baking powder
- ½ tsp ground cinnamon
- ¼ tsp erythritol

DIRECTIONS
For the custard filling:

1. In a medium bowl, beat the egg yolks with the erythritol. Mix in the xanthan gum until smooth.
2. Pour the heavy cream into a medium saucepan and simmer over low heat. Pour the mixture into the egg mixture while whisking vigorously until well mixed.
3. Transfer the mixture to the saucepan and continue whisking while cooking over low heat until thickened, 20 to 30 seconds. Turn the heat off and stir in the vanilla extract.
4. Strain the custard through a fine-mesh into a bowl. Cover the bowl with plastic wrap.
5. Refrigerate for 1 hour.

For the chaffles:

6. After 1 hour, preheat the waffle iron.
7. In a medium bowl, mix all the ingredients for the chaffles.
8. Open the iron and add a quarter of the mixture. Close and cook until crispy, 7 minutes.
9. Transfer the chaffle to a plate and make 3 more with the remaining batter.
10. To serve:
11. spread the custard filling between two chaffle quarters, sandwich and enjoy!

NUTRITION: Calories 239Fats 21.25gCarbs 3.21gNet Carbs 3.01gProtein 6.73g

78. Tiramisu Chaffles

Preparation Time: 20 minutes

Cooking Time: 28 minutes

Servings: 4

INGREDIENTS

For the chaffles:

- 2 eggs, beaten
- 3 tbsp cream cheese, softened
- ½ cup finely grated gouda cheese
- 1 tsp vanilla extract
- 1/4 tsp erythritol
- For the coffee syrup:
- 2 tbsp strong coffee, room temperature
- 3 tbsp sugar-free maple syrup

For the filling:

- ¼ cup heavy cream
- 2 tsp vanilla extract
- ¼ tsp erythritol
- 4 tbsp mascarpone cheese, room temperature
- 1 tbsp cream cheese, softened
- For dusting:
- ½ tsp unsweetened cocoa powder

DIRECTIONS
For the chaffles:

1. Preheat the waffle iron.
2. In a medium bowl, mix all the ingredients for the chaffles.
3. Open the iron and add a quarter of the mixture. Close and cook until crispy, 7 minutes.
4. Transfer the chaffle to a plate and make 3 more with the remaining batter.

For the coffee syrup:

5. In a small bowl, mix the coffee and maple syrup. Set aside.

For the filling:

6. Beat the heavy cream, vanilla, and erythritol in a medium bowl using an electric hand mixer until stiff peak forms.
7. In another bowl, beat the mascarpone cheese and cream cheese until well combined. Add the heavy cream mixture and fold in. Spoon the mixture into a piping bag.

To assemble:

8. Spoon 1 tbsp of the coffee syrup on one chaffle and pipe some of the cream cheese mixture on top. Cover with another chaffle and continue the assembling process.
9. Generously dust with cocoa powder and refrigerate overnight.
10. When ready to enjoy, slice and serve.

NUTRITION: Calories 208Fats 15.91gCarbs 4.49gNet Carbs 4.39gProtein 10.1g

79. Coconut Chaffles With Mint Frosting

Preparation Time: 15 minutes

Cooking Time: 28 minutes

Servings: 4

INGREDIENTS

For the chaffles:

- 2 eggs, beaten
- 2 tbsp cream cheese, softened

- 1 cup finely grated monterey jack cheese
- 2 tbsp coconut flour
- ¼ tsp baking powder
- 1 tbsp unsweetened shredded coconut
- 1 tbsp walnuts, chopped

For the frosting:

- ¼ cup unsalted butter, room temperature
- 3 tbsp almond milk
- 1 tsp mint extract
- 2 drops green food coloring
- 3 cups swerve confectioner's sugar

DIRECTIONS
For the chaffles:

1. Preheat the waffle iron.
2. In a medium bowl, mix all the ingredients for the chaffles.
3. Open the iron and add a quarter of the mixture. Close and cook until crispy, 7 minutes.
4. Transfer the chaffle to a plate and make 3 more with the remaining batter.

For the frosting:

5. In a medium bowl, cream the butter using an electric hand mixer until smooth.
6. Gradually mix in the almond milk until smooth.
7. Add the mint extract and green food coloring; whisk until well combined.
8. Finally, mix in the swerve confectioner's sugar a cup at a time until smooth.
9. Layer the chaffles with the frosting.
10. Slice and serve afterward.

NUTRITION: Calories 141Fats 13.13gCarbs 1.31gNet Carbs 1.03gProtein 4.31g

80. Cinnamon Roll Chaffles

Preparation Time: 15 minutes

Cooking Time: 28 minutes

Servings: 4

INGREDIENTS

For the cinnamon roll chaffles:

- ½ cup finely grated mozzarella cheese
- 1 egg, beaten
- 1 tsp cinnamon powder
- 1 tbsp almond flour
- 1 tsp erythritol

For the cinnamon roll swirl:

- 1 tbsp butter
- 1 tsp cinnamon powder
- 2 tsp erythritol

For the cinnamon roll glaze:

- 1 tbsp butter, melted
- 1 tbsp cream cheese, melted
- ¼ tsp vanilla extract
- 2 tsp swerve confectioner's sugar

DIRECTIONS

1. Preheat the waffle iron.
2. In a medium bowl, mix all the ingredients for the chaffles. Set aside.
3. In another bowl, mix all the ingredients for the cinnamon roll swirl.

4. Open the iron and lightly grease with cooking spray. Add a quarter of the chaffle mixture and top with the cinnamon roll swirl mixture.
5. Close the lid and cook until brown and crispy, 7 minutes.
6. Transfer the chaffle to a plate and make 3 more with the remaining ingredients.
7. Meanwhile, in a small bowl, whisk the glaze ingredients until smooth.
8. Drizzle the glaze over the chaffles when they are ready and serve afterward.

NUTRITION: Calories 112 Fats 10.2g Carbs 2.1g Net Carbs 1.2g Protein 3.38g

81. Chocolate Melt Chaffles

Preparation Time: 15 minutes

Cooking Time: 36 minutes

Servings: 4

INGREDIENTS

For the chaffles:

- 2 eggs, beaten
- ¼ cup finely grated gruyere cheese
- 2 tbsp heavy cream
- 1 tbsp coconut flour
- 2 tbsp cream cheese, softened
- 3 tbsp unsweetened cocoa powder
- 2 tsp vanilla extract
- A pinch of salt

For the chocolate sauce:

- 1/3 cup + 1 tbsp heavy cream
- 1 ½ oz unsweetened baking chocolate, chopped

- 1 ½ tsp sugar-free maple syrup
- 1 ½ tsp vanilla extract

DIRECTIONS
For the chaffles:

1. Preheat the waffle iron.
2. In a medium bowl, mix all the ingredients for the chaffles.
3. Open the iron and add a quarter of the mixture. Close and cook until crispy, 7 minutes.
4. Transfer the chaffle to a plate and make 3 more with the remaining batter.

For the chocolate sauce:

5. Pour the heavy cream into saucepan and simmer over low heat, 3 minutes.
6. Turn the heat off and add the chocolate. Allow melting for a few minutes and stir until fully melted, 5 minutes.
7. Mix in the maple syrup and vanilla extract.
8. Assemble the chaffles in layers with the chocolate sauce sandwiched between each layer.
9. Slice and serve immediately.

NUTRITION: Calories 172Fats 13.57gCarbs 6.65gNet Carbs 3.65gProtein 5.76g

82.   Chaffles With Keto Ice Cream

Preparation Time: 10 minutes

Cooking Time: 14 minutes

Servings: 2

INGREDIENTS

- 1 egg, beaten
- ½ cup finely grated mozzarella cheese

- ¼ cup almond flour
- 2 tbsp swerve confectioner's sugar
- 1/8 tsp xanthan gum
- Low-carb ice cream (flavor of your choice) for serving

DIRECTIONS

1. Preheat the waffle iron.
2. In a medium bowl, mix all the ingredients except the ice cream.
3. Open the iron and add half of the mixture. Close and cook until crispy, 7 minutes.
4. Transfer the chaffle to a plate and make second one with the remaining batter.
5. On each chaffle, add a scoop of low carb ice cream, fold into half-moons and enjoy.

NUTRITION: Calories 89Fats 6.48gCarbs 1.67gNet Carbs 1.37gProtein 5.91g

83.   Chicken Mozzarella Chaffle

Servings: 2

Preparation Time: 5 minutes

INGREDIENTS

- Chicken: 1 cup
- Egg: 2
- Mozzarella cheese: 1 cup and 4 tbsp
- Tomato sauce: 6 tbsp
- Basil: ½ tsp
- Garlic: ½ tbsp
- Butter: 1 tsp

DIRECTIONS

1. In a pan, add butter and include small pieces of chicken to it

2. Stir for two minutes and then add garlic and basil
3. Set aside the cooked chicken
4. Preheat the mini waffle maker if needed
5. Mix cooked chicken, eggs, and 1 cup mozzarella cheese properly
6. Spread it to the mini waffle maker thoroughly
7. Cook for 4 minutes or till it turns crispy and then remove it from the waffle maker
8. Make as many mini chaffles as you can
9. Now in a baking tray, line these mini chaffles and top with the tomato sauce and grated mozzarella cheese
10. Put the tray in the oven at 400 degrees until the cheese melts
11. Serve hot

84. Chicken Jamaican Jerk Chicken Chaffle

Servings: 2

Preparation Time: 15 minutes

INGREDIENTS

For chaffle:

- Egg: 2
- Mozzarella cheese: 1 cup (shredded)
- Butter: 1 tbsp
- Almond flour: 2 tbsp
- Turmeric: ¼ tsp
- Baking powder: ¼ tsp
- Xanthan gum: a pinch
- Onion powder: a pinch
- Garlic powder: a pinch
- Salt: a pinch

For chicken jamaican jerk:

- Organic ground chicken: 1 pound

- Dried thyme: 1 tsp
- Garlic: 1 tsp (granulated)
- Butter: 2 tbsp
- Dried parsley: 2 tsp
- Black pepper: 1/8 tsp
- Salt: 1 tsp
- Chicken broth: ½ cup
- Jerk seasoning: 2 tbsp
- Onion: ½ medium chopped

DIRECTIONS

1. In a pan, melt butter and sauté onion
2. Add all the remaining ingredients of chicken jamaican jerk and sauté
3. Now add chicken and chicken broth and stir
4. Cook on medium-low heat for 10 minutes
5. Then cook on high heat and dry all the liquid
6. For chaffles, preheat a mini waffle maker if needed and grease it
7. In a mixing bowl, beat all the chaffle ingredients
8. Pour the mixture to the lower plate of the waffle maker and spread it evenly to cover the plate properly and close the lid
9. Cook for at least 4 minutes to get the desired crunch
10. Remove the chaffle from the heat and keep aside for around one minute
11. Make as many chaffles as your mixture and waffle maker allow
12. Add the chicken in between of a chaffle and fold and enjoy

85.   Chicken Green Chaffles

Servings: 4

Preparation Time: 10 minutes

INGREDIENTS

For chaffle:

- Chicken: 1/3 cup boiled and shredded
- Cabbage: 1/3 cup
- Broccoli: 1/3 cup
- Zucchini: 1/3 cup
- Egg: 2
- Mozzarella cheese: 1 cup (shredded)
- Butter: 1 tbsp
- Almond flour: 2 tbsp
- Baking powder: ¼ tsp
- onion powder: a pinch
- garlic powder: a pinch
- salt: a pinch

DIRECTIONS

1. In a deep saucepan, boil cabbage, broccoli, and zucchini for five minutes or till it tenders, strain, and blend
2. Mix all the remaining ingredients well together
3. Pour a thin layer on a preheated waffle iron
4. Add a layer of the blended vegetables on the mixture
5. again add more mixture over the top
6. Cook the chaffle for around 5 minutes
7. Serve with your favorite sauce

SNACKS

86.   Vanilla Raspberry Chaffle

Preparation Time: 5 minutes

Cooking Time: 8 minutes

Servings: 2

INGREDIENTS

- ½ cup cream cheese, soft
- 1 teaspoon vanilla extract
- 1 tablespoon almond flour
- ¼ cup raspberries, pureed
- 1 egg, whisked
- 1 tablespoon monk fruit

DIRECTIONS

1. In a bowl, mix the cream cheese with the raspberry puree and the other ingredients and whisk well.
2. Heat up the waffle iron over high heat, pour half of the batter, close the waffle maker, cook for 8 minutes and transfer to a plate.
3. Repeat with the rest of the batter and servings the chaffles warm.

NUTRITION: Calories 150, Fat 9.3, Fiber 1.2, Carbs 3.4, Protein 4.2

87.   Nutmeg Chaffle

Preparation Time: 5 minutes

Cooking Time: 5 minutes

Servings: 2

INGREDIENTS

- 3 tablespoons heavy cream
- 1 tablespoon coconut oil, melted
- 1 tablespoon coconut flour
- 1 egg, whisked
- 1 tablespoon stevia
- ½ teaspoon nutmeg, ground
- 2 tablespoons cream cheese
- ½ teaspoon vanilla extract

DIRECTIONS

1. In a bowl, mix the cream with the coconut oil, egg and the other ingredients and whisk well.
2. Heat up the waffle iron over high heat, pour half of the batter, close the waffle maker, cook for 5 minutes and transfer to a plate.
3. Repeat with the remaining batter and servings.

NUTRITION: Calories 200, Fat 15, Fiber 1.2, Carbs 3.4, Protein 12.05

88. Almond Plums Chaffle

Preparation Time: 5 minutes

Cooking Time: 6 minutes

Servings: 4

INGREDIENTS

- ½ cup heavy cream
- ½ cup almonds, chopped
- 2 plums, pitted and chopped
- 1 tablespoon almond flour

- 3 eggs, whisked
- 2 tablespoons erythritol
- 2 tablespoons cream cheese

DIRECTIONS

1. In a bowl, mix the cream with the almonds, plums and the other ingredients and whisk well.
2. Heat up the waffle iron over high heat, pour ¼ of the batter, close the waffle maker, cook for 6 minutes and transfer to a plate.
3. Repeat with the remaining batter and servings the chaffles warm.

NUTRITION: Calories 220, Fat 13.25, Fiber 1.2, Carbs 5.4, Protein 12

89.   <u>Almond Butter Chaffle</u>

Preparation Time: 5 minutes

Cooking Time: 6 minutes

Servings: 4

INGREDIENTS

- 4 eggs, whisked
- 1 cup almond flour
- 2 tablespoons swerve
- ½ cup almond butter, soft
- 1 teaspoon baking soda
- 2 teaspoons vanilla extract
- 2 tablespoons coconut oil, melted

DIRECTIONS

1. In a bowl, combine the eggs with the almond flour, swerve and the other ingredients and whisk well.

2. Heat up the waffle iron over high heat, pour ¼ of the batter, close the waffle maker, cook for 6 minutes and transfer to a plate.
3. Repeat with the rest batter and servings the chaffles warm.

NUTRITION: Calories 220, Fat 4.3, Fiber 1.2, Carbs 3.4, Protein 7.5

90. Mint Chaffle

Preparation Time: 5 minutes

Cooking Time: 5 minutes

Servings: 2

INGREDIENTS

- ½ cup cream cheese, soft
- 1 tablespoon almond flour
- ½ tablespoon coconut flour
- 2 eggs whisked
- 1 tablespoon swerve
- 2 tablespoons mint, chopped
- 1 teaspoon vanilla extract
- ½ teaspoon almond extract

DIRECTIONS

1. In a bowl, combine the cream cheese with the flour and the other ingredients and whisk well.
2. Heat up the waffle iron over high heat, pour half of the batter, close the waffle maker, cook for 5 minutes and transfer to a plate.
3. Repeat with the other part of the batter and servings the chaffles warm.

NUTRITION: Calories 182, Fat 8.3, Fiber 1.2, Carbs 3.4, Protein 6.5

91. Melon Puree Chaffle

Preparation Time: 5 minutes

Cooking Time: 5 minutes

Servings: 2

INGREDIENTS

- ½ cup melon, peeled and pureed
- 3 tablespoons cream cheese, soft
- 1 tablespoon coconut flour
- 1 egg, whisked
- 1 tablespoon stevia
- ½ teaspoon almond extract

DIRECTIONS

1. In a bowl, mix the melon puree with the cream cheese and the other ingredients and whisk well.
2. Heat up the waffle iron over high heat, pour half of the batter, close the waffle maker, cook for 5 minutes and transfer to a plate.
3. Repeat with the other part of the batter and servings.

NUTRITION: Calories 252, Fat 14.3, Fiber 3.2, Carbs 4.4, Protein 2.3

92. Sweet Zucchini Chaffle

Preparation Time: 5 minutes

Cooking Time: 7 minutes

Servings: 4

INGREDIENTS

- ½ cup zucchinis, grated
- 4 tablespoons cream cheese, soft
- 1 tablespoon almond flour
- 1 tablespoon almonds, chopped
- 2 eggs, whisked
- 1 tablespoon swerve
- ½ teaspoon vanilla extract

DIRECTIONS

1. In a bowl, mix the zucchinis with the cream cheese, almond flour and other ingredients and whisk well.
2. Heat up the waffle iron over high heat, pour ¼ of the batter, close the waffle maker, cook for 7 minutes and transfer to a plate.
3. Repeat with the remaining batter and servings the chaffles hot.

NUTRITION: Calories 220, Fat 12.4, Fiber 2.2, Carbs 3.4, Protein 6.4

93.   Pumpkin and Avocado Chaffle

Preparation Time: 5 minutes

Cooking Time: 5 minutes

Servings: 4

INGREDIENTS

- ½ cup heavy cream
- 1 avocado, peeled, pitted and mashed
- 1 tablespoon coconut flour
- 2 eggs, whisked
- 2 tablespoons swerve
- 2 and ½ tablespoons pumpkin puree

- 2 tablespoons cream cheese, soft

DIRECTIONS

1. In a bowl, combine the cream with the avocado, pumpkin puree and the other ingredients and whisk.
2. Heat up the waffle iron over high heat, pour ¼ of the batter, close the waffle maker, cook for 5 minutes and transfer to a plate.
3. Repeat with the rest of the batter and servings the chaffles warm.

NUTRITION: Calories 220, Fat 9.4, Fiber 1.2, Carbs 3, Protein 7.6

94.   Nuts chaffle

Preparation Time: 5 minutes

Cooking Time: 8 minutes

Servings: 4

INGREDIENTS

- 2 tablespoons almonds, chopped
- 2 tablespoons walnuts, chopped
- 1 tablespoon stevia
- ½ cup cream cheese, soft
- 2 eggs, whisked
- 1 tablespoon almond flour
- 1 tablespoon coconut flour
- ½ teaspoon almond extract

DIRECTIONS

1. In a blender, mix the almonds with the walnuts, cream cheese and the other ingredients and pulse well.

2. Heat up the waffle iron over high heat, pour ¼ of the batter, close the waffle maker, cook for 5 minutes and transfer to a plate.
3. Repeat with the other part of the batter and servings.

NUTRITION: Calories 200, Fat 9.34, Fiber 2.2, Carbs 4.4, Protein 8.4

95. Blueberries and Almonds Chaffles

Preparation Time: 5 minutes

Cooking Time: 8 minutes

Servings: 6

INGREDIENTS

- ½ cup cream cheese, soft
- ½ cup blueberries pureed
- 2 tablespoons almonds
- 1 tablespoon almond flour
- 2 eggs, whisked
- 1 and ½ tablespoon stevia
- ½ teaspoon almond extract

DIRECTIONS

1. In a bowl, mix the cream cheese with the blueberries, eggs and the other ingredients and whisk well.
2. Heat up the waffle iron over high heat, pour 1/6 of the batter, close the waffle maker, cook for 5 minutes and transfer to a plate.
3. Repeat with the other part of the batter and servings.

NUTRITION: Calories 180, Fat 5.4, Fiber 1.2, Carbs 2.24, Protein 2.4

96. Rhubarb Chaffles

Preparation Time: 5 minutes

Cooking Time: 6 minutes

Servings: 3

INGREDIENTS

- ½ cup rhubarb, chopped
- ¼ cup heavy cream
- 3 tablespoons cream cheese, soft
- 2 tablespoons almond flour
- 2 eggs, whisked
- 2 tablespoons swerve
- ½ teaspoon vanilla extract
- ½ teaspoon nutmeg, ground

DIRECTIONS

1. In a bowl, mix the rhubarb with the cream, cream cheese and the other ingredients and whisk well.
2. Heat up the waffle iron over high heat, pour 1/3 of the batter, close the waffle maker, cook for 5 minutes and transfer to a plate.
3. Repeat with the rest of the chaffle batter and servings.

NUTRITION: Calories 180, Fat 4, Fiber 1.2, Carbs 2, Protein 2.4

97. Sweet Turmeric Chaffles

Preparation Time: 5 minutes

Cooking Time: 6 minutes

Servings: 2

INGREDIENTS

- 3 tablespoons cream cheese, soft
- ½ teaspoon turmeric powder
- ½ teaspoon vanilla extract
- 2 tablespoons coconut flour
- 2 eggs, whisked
- 2 tablespoons stevia

DIRECTIONS

1. In a bowl, mix the cream cheese with the turmeric, vanilla and the other ingredients and whisk well.
2. Heat up the waffle iron over high heat, pour ½ of the batter, close the waffle maker, cook for 6 minutes and transfer to a plate.
3. Repeat with the other part of the batter and servings right away.

NUTRITION: Calories 140, Fat 4.4, Fiber 1.2, Carbs 5.4, Protein 4.4

98. Banana Pudding Chaffle Cake

PREPARATION Time: 5 minutes

Cooking Time: 5 minutes

Servings: 2

INGREDIENTS

- 1 large egg yolk
- 1/2 cup fresh cream
- 3 t powder sweetener
- 1 4-1 2 teaspoon xanthan gum
- 1/2 teaspoon banana extract

Banana chaffle ingredients

- 1 oz softened cream cheese
- 1/4 cup mozzarella cheese shredded
- 1 egg
- 1 teaspoon banana extract
- 2 t sweetener
- 1 tsp baking powder
- 4 t almond flour

PREPARATIONS

1. Mix heavy cream, powdered sweetener and egg yolk in a small pot. Whisk constantly until the sweetener has dissolved and the mixture is thick.
2. Cook for 1 minute. Add xanthan gum and whisk.
3. Remove from heat, add a pinch of salt and banana extract and stir well.
4. Transfer to a glass dish and cover the pudding with plastic wrap. Refrigerate.
5. Mix all ingredients together. Cook in a preheated mini waffle maker.

Note: Make three chaffles. 3.3 net Carbs / serving. Recipe 9.8 net Carbs Nutrition

99.   Maple Pumpkin Keto Chaffle

Preparation Time: 5 minutes

Cooking Time: 4 minutes

Servings: 2

INGREDIENTS

- 3/4 tsp baking powder
- 2 eggs
- 4 tsp heavy whipping cream

- 1/2 cup mozzarella cheese, shredded
- 2 tsp liquid stevia
- Pinch of salt
- 3/4 tsp pumpkin pie spice
- 1 tsp coconut flour
- 2 tsp pumpkin puree (100% pumpkin)
- 1/2 tsp vanilla

DIRECTIONS

1. Preheat mini waffle maker until hot
2. Whisk egg in a bowl, add cheese, then mix well
3. Stir in the remaining ingredients (except toppings, if any).
4. Scoop 1/2 of the batter onto the waffle maker, spread across evenly
5. Cook 3-4 minutes, until done as desired (or crispy).
6. Gently remove from waffle maker and let it cool
7. Repeat with remaining batter.
8. Top with sugar-free maple syrup or keto ice cream.
9. Servings and enjoy!

NUTRITION: 201 Calories 2g net Carbs 15g Fat 12g Protein

100. Keto Almond Blueberry Chaffle

Preparation Time: 5 minutes

Cooking Time: 5 minutes

Servings: 5 chaffles

INGREDIENTS

- 1 tsp baking powder
- 2 eggs
- 1 cup of mozzarella cheese
- 2 tablespoons almond flour
- 3 tablespoon blueberries

- 1 tsp cinnamon
- 2 tsp of swerve

DIRECTIONS

1. Preheat mini waffle maker until hot
2. Whisk egg in a bowl, add cheese, then mix well
3. Stir in the remaining ingredients (except toppings, if any).
4. Grease the preheated waffle maker with non-stick cooking spray.
5. Scoop 1/2 of the batter onto the waffle maker, spread across evenly
6. Cook until a bit browned and crispy, about 4 minutes.
7. Cook 3-4 minutes, until done as desired (or crispy).
8. Gently remove from waffle maker and let it cool
9. Repeat with remaining batter.
10. Top with keto syrup
11. Servings and enjoy!

NUTRITION: 116 Calories 1g net Carbs 8g Fat 8g Protein

DESSERT

101. Sweet Cinnamon "Sugar" Chaffle

Preparation Time: 5 minutes

Cooking Time: 4 minutes

Servings: 1

INGREDIENTS

- 1/2 teaspoon cinnamon (topping)
- 10 drops of liquid stevia
- 1 tablespoon almond flour
- Two large eggs
- A splash of vanilla
- 1/2 cup mozzarella cheese

DIRECTIONS

1. Preheat waffle maker until hot
2. Whisk egg in a bowl, add cheese, then mix well
3. Stir in the remaining ingredients (except toppings, if any).
4. Scoop 1/2 of the batter onto the waffle maker, spread across evenly
5. Cook 3-4 minutes, until done as desired (or crispy).
6. Gently remove from waffle maker and let it cool
7. Repeat with remaining batter.
8. Top with melted butter and sprinkle of cinnamon.
9. Servings and enjoy!

NUTRITION: 221 Calories 2g net Carbs 17g Fat 12g Protein

102. Chocolatey Chaffle

Preparation Time: 5 minutes

Cooking Time: 4 minutes

Servings: 2

INGREDIENTS

- 1 large egg
- 1 oz. Cream cheese, softened
- 1 tbsp choczero chocolate syrup
- 1/2 tsp vanilla
- 1 tbsp stevia sweetener
- 1/2 tbsp cacao powder
- 1/4 tsp baking powder

DIRECTIONS

1. Preheat mini waffle maker until hot
2. Whisk egg in a bowl, add cheese, then mix well
3. Stir in the remaining ingredients (except toppings, if any).
4. Scoop 1/2 of the batter onto the waffle maker, spread across evenly
5. Cook until a bit browned and crispy, about 4 minutes.
6. Gently remove from waffle maker and let it cool
7. Repeat with remaining batter.
8. Servings and enjoy!

NUTRITION: 241 Calories 2g net Carbs 19g Fat 13g Protein

103. <u>Keto Chocolate Chip Chaffle</u>

Preparation Time: 5 minutes

Cooking Time: 8 minutes

Servings: 1

INGREDIENTS

- 1 egg

- 1/4 tsp baking powder
- pinch of salt
- 1 tbsp heavy whipping cream (topping)
- 1/2 tsp coconut flour
- 1 tbsp chocolate chips

DIRECTIONS

1. Preheat mini waffle maker until hot
2. Whisk egg in a bowl, add cheese, then mix well
3. Stir in the remaining ingredients (except toppings, if any).
4. Grease preheated waffle maker with. This will help to create a crisper crust.
5. Scoop 1/2 of the batter onto the waffle maker, spread across evenly.
6. Sprinkle chocolate chips on top
7. Cook until a bit browned and crispy, about 4 minutes.
8. Gently remove from waffle maker and let it cool
9. Repeat with remaining batter.
10. Top with whipping cream
11. Servings and enjoy!

NUTRITION: 146 Calories 3g net Carbs 10g Fat 6g Protein

104. Pumpkin Chocolate Chip Chaffles

Preparation Time: 4 minutes

Cooking Time: 12 minutes

Servings: 3

INGREDIENTS

- 2 tbsp granulated swerve
- 1/4 tsp pumpkin pie spice
- 1 tbsp almond flour
- 1/2 cup shredded mozzarella cheese
- 4 tsp pumpkin puree

- 1 egg
- 4 tsp chocolate chips

DIRECTIONS

1. Preheat mini waffle maker until hot
2. Whisk egg in a bowl, add cheese, then mix well
3. Stir in the remaining ingredients (except toppings, if any).
4. Grease waffle maker and scoop 1/2 of the batter onto the waffle maker, spread across evenly.
5. Add chocolate chips on top the batter and cook until a bit browned and crispy, about 4 minutes.
6. Gently remove from waffle maker and let it cool
7. Repeat with remaining batter.
8. Servings and enjoy with some cream!

NUTRITION: 93 Calories 1g net Carbs 7g Fat 7g Protein

105.   Mint Chocolate Chaffle

Preparation Time: 5 minutes

Cooking Time: 4 minutes

Servings: 2

INGREDIENTS

- 1 large egg
- 1 oz. Cream cheese, softened
- 1 tbsp chocolate chips
- 1 tbsp stevia sweetener
- 1 tbsp low carb mint extract
- 1/2 tbsp cacao powder
- 1/4 tsp baking powder

DIRECTIONS

1. Preheat mini waffle maker until hot

2. Whisk egg in a bowl, add cheese, then mix well
3. Stir in the remaining ingredients (except toppings, if any).
4. Scoop 1/2 of the batter onto the waffle maker, spread across evenly
5. Cook until a bit browned and crispy, about 4 minutes.
6. Gently remove from waffle maker and let it cool
7. Repeat with remaining batter.
8. Servings and enjoy!

NUTRITION: 241 Calories 2g net Carbs 19g Fat 13g Protein

106.   Keto Coco-Chaffle

Preparation Time: 5 minutes

Cooking Time: 8 minutes

Servings: 1

INGREDIENTS

- 1 egg
- 1/4 tsp baking powder
- Pinch of salt
- 1 tbsp heavy whipping cream (topping)
- 1/2 tsp coconut flour
- 1 tbsp chocolate chips

DIRECTIONS

1. Preheat mini waffle maker until hot
2. Whisk egg in a bowl, add cheese, then mix well
3. Stir in the remaining ingredients (except toppings, if any).
4. Grease preheated waffle maker with non-stick cooking spray. Scoop 1/2 of the batter onto the waffle maker, spread across evenly.
5. Sprinkle cocoa powder on top
6. Cook until a bit browned and crispy, about 4 minutes.

7. Gently remove from waffle maker and let it cool
8. Repeat with remaining batter.
9. Top with whipping cream
10. Servings and enjoy!

NUTRITION: 146 Calories 3g net Carbs 10g Fat 6g Protein

107. <u>Keto Vanilla Brownie Chaffle</u>

Preparation Time: 5 minutes

Cooking Time: 4 minutes

Servings: 2

INGREDIENTS

- 1 large egg
- 1 oz. Cream cheese, softened
- 1 tbsp choczero chocolate syrup
- 1/2 tsp vanilla
- 2 tbsp stevia sweetener
- 2 tbsp cacao powder
- 1/4 tsp baking powder

DIRECTIONS

1. Preheat mini waffle maker until hot
2. Whisk egg in a bowl, add cheese, then mix well
3. Stir in the remaining ingredients (except toppings, if any).
4. Scoop 1/2 of the batter onto the waffle maker, spread across evenly
5. Cook until a bit browned and crispy, about 4 minutes.
6. Gently remove from waffle maker and let it cool
7. Repeat with remaining batter.
8. Servings and enjoy with topped melted butter!

NUTRITION: 241 Calories 2g net Carbs 19g Fat 13g Protein

108. Keto Crispy Choco Chaffle

Preparation Time: 5 minutes

Cooking Time: 8 minutes

Servings: 1

INGREDIENTS

- 1 egg
- 1/4 tsp baking powder
- Pinch of salt
- 1 tbsp almond butter (topping)
- 1/2 tsp almond flour
- 1 tbsp chocolate chips
- 1 tsp cheddar cheese (servings ½ for greasing)

DIRECTIONS

1. Preheat mini waffle maker until hot
2. Whisk egg in a bowl, add cheese, then mix well
3. Stir in the remaining ingredients (except toppings, if any).
4. Grease preheated waffle maker with 1 tsp of shredded cheese. Cook for 20 seconds. This will help to create a more crisp crust.
5. Scoop 1/2 of the batter onto the waffle maker, spread across evenly.
6. Sprinkle chocolate chips on top
7. Cook until a bit browned and crispy, about 4 minutes.
8. Gently remove from waffle maker and let it cool
9. Repeat with remaining batter.
10. Top with whipping cream
11. Servings and enjoy!

NUTRITION: 146 Calories 3g net Carbs 10g Fat 6g Protein

109. Almond Chocolate Chaffle

Preparation Time: 5 minutes

Cooking Time: 4 minutes

Servings: 2

INGREDIENTS

- 1 large egg
- 1 oz. Cream cheese, softened
- 1 tbsp choczero chocolate syrup
- 1/2 tsp vanilla
- 1 tbsp stevia sweetener
- 1/2 tbsp cacao powder
- 1/4 tsp baking powder
- One handful almond nuts, cut in bit sizes (topping)

DIRECTIONS

1. Preheat mini waffle maker until hot
2. Whisk egg in a bowl, add cheese, then mix well
3. Stir in the remaining ingredients (except toppings).
4. Scoop 1/2 of the batter onto the waffle maker, spread across evenly
5. Sprinkle almond nuts, then cover and cook until a bit browned and crispy, about 4 minutes.
6. Gently remove from waffle maker and let it cool
7. Repeat with remaining batter.
8. Servings and enjoy!

NUTRITION: 241 Calories 2g net Carbs 19g Fat 13g Protein

110. Keto Chocolate Chip Chaffle

Preparation Time: 5 minutes

Cooking Time: 8 minutes

Servings: 1

INGREDIENTS

- 1 egg
- 1/4 tsp baking powder
- Pinch of salt
- 1 tbsp cinnamon (topping)
- 1/2 tsp coconut flour
- 1 tbsp chocolate chips

DIRECTIONS

1. Preheat mini waffle maker until hot
2. Whisk egg in a bowl, add cheese, then mix well
3. Stir in the remaining ingredients (except toppings, if any).
4. Grease preheated waffle maker with. This will help to create a crisper crust.
5. Scoop 1/2 of the batter onto the waffle maker, spread across evenly.
6. Sprinkle chocolate chips on top
7. Cook until a bit browned and crispy, about 4 minutes.
8. Gently remove from waffle maker and let it cool
9. Repeat with remaining batter.
10. Top with whipping cream
11. Servings and enjoy!

NUTRITION: 146 Calories 3g net Carbs 10g Fat 6g Protein

111.   Sweet Raspberry Chaffle

Preparation Time: 5 minutes

Cooking Time: 5 minutes

Servings: 5 chaffles

INGREDIENTS

- 1 tsp baking powder
- 2 eggs
- 1 cup of mozzarella cheese
- 2 tbsp almond flour
- 4 raspberries, chopped
- 1 tsp cinnamon
- 10 drops stevia, liquid

DIRECTIONS

1. Preheat mini waffle maker until hot
2. Whisk egg in a bowl, add cheese, then mix well
3. Stir in the remaining ingredients (except toppings, if any).
4. Grease the preheated waffle maker with non-stick cooking spray.
5. Scoop 1/2 of the batter onto the waffle maker, spread across evenly
6. Cook until a bit browned and crispy, about 4 minutes.
7. Cook 3-4 minutes, until done as desired (or crispy).
8. Gently remove from waffle maker and let it cool
9. Repeat with remaining batter.
10. Top with keto syrup
11. Servings and enjoy!

NUTRITION: 116 Calories 1g net Carbs 8g Fat 8g Protein

112. Keto Ice-Cream Chaffle

Servings: 2

Preparation Time: 15 minutes

INGREDIENTS

- Egg: 1
- Swerve/monkfruit: 2 tbsp
- Baking powder: 1 tbsp

- Heavy whipping cream: 1 tbsp
- Keto ice cream: as per your choice

DIRECTIONS

1. Take a small bowl and whisk the egg and add all the ingredients
2. Beat until the mixture becomes creamy
3. Pour the mixture to the lower plate of the waffle maker and spread it evenly to cover the plate properly
4. Close the lid
5. Cook for at least 4 minutes to get the desired crunch
6. Remove the chaffle from the heat and keep aside for a few minutes
7. Make as many chaffles as your mixture and waffle maker allow
8. Top with your favorite ice cream and enjoy!

113. Double Chocolate Chaffle

Servings: 2

Preparation Time: 5 minutes

INGREDIENTS

- Egg: 2
- Coconut flour: 4 tbsp
- Cocoa powder: 2 tbsp
- Cream cheese: 2 oz
- Baking powder: ½ tsp
- Chocolate chips: 2 tbsp (unsweetened)
- Vanilla extract: 1 tsp
- Swerve/monkfruit: 4 tbsp

DIRECTIONS

1. Preheat a mini waffle maker if needed and grease it
2. In a mixing bowl, beat eggs

3. In a separate mixing bowl, add coconut flour, cocoa powder, swerve/monkfruit, and baking powder, when combine pour into eggs with cream cheese and vanilla extracts
4. Mix them all well to give them uniform consistency and pour the mixture to the lower plate of the waffle maker
5. On top of the mixture, sprinkle around half tsp of unsweetened chocolate chips and close the lid
6. Cook for at least 4 minutes to get the desired crunch
7. Remove the chaffle from the heat and keep aside for around one minute
8. Make as many chaffles as your mixture and waffle maker allow
9. Serve with your favorite whipped cream or berries

114. Cream Cheese Mini Chaffle

Servings: 2

Preparation Time: 5 minutes

INGREDIENTS

- Egg: 1
- Coconut flour: 2 tbsp
- Cream cheese: 1 oz
- Baking powder: ¼ tsp
- Vanilla extract: ½ tsp
- Swerve/monkfruit: 4 tsp

DIRECTIONS

1. Preheat a waffle maker if needed and grease it
2. In a mixing bowl, mix coconut flour, swerve/monkfruit, and baking powder
3. Now add an egg to the mixture with cream cheese and vanilla extract
4. Mix them all well and pour the mixture to the lower plate of the waffle maker
5. Close the lid

6. Cook for at least 4 minutes to get the desired crunch
7. Remove the chaffle from the heat
8. Make as many chaffles as your mixture and waffle maker allow
9. Eat the chaffles with your favorite toppings

115. Choco Chip Cannoli Chaffle

Servings: 4

Preparation Time: 10 minutes

INGREDIENTS

For chaffle:

- Egg yolk: 1
- Swerve/monkfruit: 1 tbsp
- Baking powder: 1/8 tbsp
- Vanilla extract: 1/8 tsp
- Almond flour: 3 tbsp
- Chocolate chips: 1 tbsp

For cannoli topping:

- Cream cheese: 4 tbsp
- Ricotta: 6 tbsp
- Sweetener: 2 tbsp
- Vanilla extract: 1/4 tsp
- Lemon extract: 5 drops

DIRECTIONS

1. Preheat a mini waffle maker if needed and grease it
2. In a mixing bowl, add all the chaffle ingredients and mix well
3. Pour the mixture to the lower plate of the waffle maker and spread it evenly to cover the plate properly and close the lid

4. Cook for at least 4 minutes to get the desired crunch
5. In the meanwhile, prepare cannoli topping by adding all the ingredients in the blender to give the creamy texture
6. Remove the chaffle from the heat and keep aside to cool them down
7. Make as many chaffles as your mixture and waffle maker allow
8. Serve with the cannoli toppings and enjoy

116. Cream Cheese Pumpkin Chaffle

Servings: 2

Preparation Time: 5 minutes

INGREDIENTS

- Egg: 2
- Cream cheese: 2 oz
- Coconut flour: 2 tsp
- Swerve/monkfruit: 4 tsp
- Baking powder: ½ tsp
- Vanilla extract: 1 tsp
- Canned pumpkin: 2 tbsp
- Pumpkin spice: ½ tsp

DIRECTIONS

1. Take a small mixing bowl and add swerve/monkfruit, coconut flour, and baking powder and mix them all well
2. Now add egg, vanilla extract, pumpkin, and cream cheese, and beat them all together till uniform consistency is achieved
3. Preheat a mini waffle maker if needed
4. Pour the mixture to the greasy waffle maker
5. Cook for at least 4 minutes to get the desired crunch
6. Remove the chaffle from the heat
7. Make as many chaffles as your mixture and waffle maker allow
8. Serve with butter or whipped cream that you like!

117. Easy Blueberry Chaffle

Servings: 2

Preparation Time: 5 minutes

INGREDIENTS

- Egg: 2
- Cream cheese: 2 oz
- Coconut flour: 2 tbsp
- Swerve/monkfruit: 4 tsp
- Baking powder: ½ tsp
- Vanilla extract: 1 tsp
- Blueberries: ½ cup

DIRECTIONS

1. Take a small mixing bowl and add swerve/monkfruit, baking powder, and coconut flour and mix them all well
2. Now add eggs, vanilla extract, and cream cheese, and beat them all together till uniform consistency is achieved
3. Preheat a mini waffle maker if needed and grease it
4. Pour the mixture to the lower plate of the waffle maker
5. Add 3-4 fresh blueberries above the mixture and close the lid
6. Cook for at least 4 minutes to get the desired crunch
7. Remove the chaffle from the heat
8. Make as many chaffles as your mixture and waffle maker allow
9. Serve with butter or whipped cream that you like!

118. Apple Pie Chayote Tacos Chaffle

Servings: 2

Preparation Time: 15 minutes

INGREDIENTS

For chaffle:

- Egg: 2
- Cream cheese: ½ cup
- Baking powder: 1 tsp
- Vanilla extract: ½ tsp
- Powdered sweetener: 2 tbsp

For apple pie chayote filling:

- Chayote squash: 1
- Butter: 1 tbsp
- Swerve: ¼ cup
- Cinnamon powder: 2 tsp
- Lemon: 2 tbsp
- Cream of tartar: 1/8 tsp
- Nutmeg: 1/8 tsp
- Ginger powder: 1/8 tsp

DIRECTIONS

1. For around 25 minutes, boil the whole chayote; when it cools, peel it and slice
2. Add all the remaining filling ingredients to it
3. Bake the chayote for 20 minutes covered with foil
4. Pour ¼ of the mixtures to the blender to make it a sauce
5. Add to chayote slices and mix
6. For the chaffles, preheat a mini waffle maker if needed and grease it
7. In a mixing bowl, add all the chaffle ingredients and mix well
8. Pour the mixture to the lower plate of the waffle maker and spread it evenly to cover the plate properly and close the lid
9. Cook for at least 4 minutes to get the desired crunch
10. Make as many chaffles as your mixture and waffle maker allow

11. Fold the chaffles and serve with the chayote sauce in between

119. Rice Krispie Treat Copycat Chaffle:

Servings: 2

Preparation Time: 15 minutes

INGREDIENTS

For chaffle:

- Egg: 1
- Cream cheese: 4 tbsp
- Baking powder: 1 tsp
- Vanilla extract: ½ tsp
- Powdered sweetener: 2 tbsp
- Pork rinds: 4 tbsp (crushed)
- For marshmallow frosting:
- Heavy whipping cream: ¼ cup
- Xanthan gum: ½ tsp
- Powdered sweetener: 1 tbsp
- Vanilla extract: ¼ tsp

DIRECTIONS

1. Preheat a mini waffle maker if needed and grease it
2. In a mixing bowl, add all the chaffle ingredients
3. Mix them all well
4. Pour the mixture to the lower plate of the waffle maker and spread it evenly to cover the plate properly and close the lid
5. Cook for at least 4 minutes to get the desired crunch
6. Remove the chaffle from the heat and keep aside for around one minute
7. Make as many chaffles as your mixture and waffle maker allow

8. For the marshmallow frosting, add all the frosting ingredients except xanthan gum and whip to form a thick consistency
9. Add xanthan gum at the end and fold
10. Serve frosting with chaffles and enjoy!

120. Smores Keto Chaffle:

Servings: 2

Preparation Time: 15 minutes

INGREDIENTS

- Egg: 1
- Mozzarella cheese: ½ cup (shredded)
- Baking powder: ¼ tsp
- Vanilla extract: ½ tsp
- Swerve: 2 tbsp
- Pink salt: a pinch
- Psyllium husk powder: ½ tbsp
- Dark chocolate bar: ¼
- Keto marshmallow crème fluff: 2 tbsp

DIRECTIONS

1. Create the keto marshmallow crème fluff
2. Beat the egg that much that it will become creamy and further add swerve brown and vanilla to it and mix well
3. Now add cheese to the mixture with psyllium husk powder, salt, and baking powder and leave chocolate and marshmallow
4. Mix them all well and allow the batter to set for 3-4 minutes
5. Preheat a mini waffle maker if needed and grease it
6. Pour the mixture to the lower plate of the waffle maker and spread it evenly to cover the plate properly
7. Close the lid
8. Cook for at least 4 minutes to get the desired crunch

9. Remove the chaffle from the heat and keep aside for around one minute
10. Make as many chaffles as your mixture and waffle maker allow
11. Now serve the chaffle with 2 tbsp marshmallow and chocolate bar

OTHER KETO CHAFFLES RECIPES

121. <u>Corndog Chaffle</u>

Preparation Time: 5 minutes

Cooking Time: 5 minutes

Servings: 3

INGREDIENTS

- Mix flax egg-1 t ground flax seed with 3 t water
- If you are not allergic to egg whites, skip flax and use one large egg
- 1 1/2 t melted butter
- 2 teaspoons sweetener
- 3 t almond flour
- 1/4 teaspoon baking powder
- 1 egg yolk
- 2 t heap mexican blended cheese
- 1 t chopped jalapeno
- 15-20 drop cornbread flavor
- Extra cheese to sprinkle on waffle maker

PREPARATION

1. Mix everything together. Rest for 5 minutes. If too thick, add 1 t water or hwc.
2. Sprinkle the shredded cheese on the bottom of the waffle maker. Add 1/3 of the batter. Sprinkle the shredded cheese on top. Close the waffle iron. Do not press. If the cheese is crispy, remove it. Repeat. Make 3
3. Note: this is the cornbread flavor i used.
4. Corn silk (zea mays) glycerite, organic dry silk alcohol free liquid extract 2 oz

122. Keto Chaffle Churro

Preparation Time: 10 minutes

Cooking Time: 4 minutes

Servings: 2

INGREDIENTS

- 1 egg
- 1/2 cup mozzarella cheese shredded
- 2 tbsp swallow brown sweetener
- 1/2 tsp cinnamon

DIRECTIONS

1. Preheat the mini waffle of iron.
2. Whip the egg with a fork in a small bowl.
3. Apply the shredded cheese to the combination of eggs.
4. Place half of the egg mixture in a mini waffle pan and cook until golden brown (about 4 minutes) while the mini chaffle is cooking, add the swerve brown sweetener and cinnamon in a separate small bowl.
5. Once the chaffle is done, cut it into slices (as shown in the vacuum while it's still hot and add it to the cinnamon mixture. It soaks up more of the mixture when it's still hot! Serve warm and enjoy!

NUTRITION: Calories 76, total Fat 4.3g, cholesterol 14mg, sodium 147.5mg, total carbohydrate 4.1g, dietary Fiber 1.2g, sugars 1.9g, Protein 5.5g, vitamin a 55μg, vitamin c 0.9mg

123. Everything Chaffle

Preparation Time: 8 minutes

Cooking Time: 10 minutes

Servings: 2

INGREDIENTS

- 1 large egg
- 1 ounce 6 cheese italian blend cheese, finely shredded
- 3 tablespoons almond flour
- 1 pinch salt
- Butter flavored non-stick cooking spray

Topping

- 2 ounces cream cheese
- 2 teaspoons everything bagel seasoning

DIRECTIONS

1. Plug in the mini waffle maker and preheat it. There is a light for many waffle makers to indicate when it is preheated. Be sure that it is completely heated before continuing for the best results.
2. Crack the large egg into a small bowl and beat vigorously with a fork until well mixed yolk and white.
3. Chop the shredded italian cheese into smaller pieces using a small chopping board and medium-sized knife. It ensures that the cheese can be distributed more evenly throughout the egg mixture.
4. Add the egg mixture with the butter, almond flour and salt and whisk with a fork until all is well mixed.
5. Sprinkle waffle maker with non-stick cooking spray flavored with butter.
6. Put 1/2 of the mixture in a miniature waffle maker's grill center. Stretch the mixture to the grill edges and close the waffle maker.
7. Cook the chaffle for 5 minutes or brown and cook through until toasty.
8. Gently remove the chaffle using a small fork and place it to cool on a sheet of paper towels.
9. Spray waffle maker with non-stick cooking spray flavored with butter and cook the remaining mixture of the chaffle the same as the first.
10. When they cool down, chaffles will become crisper.

11. Layer cream cheese chaffles and sprinkle with bagel seasoning.

NUTRITION: Calories 249kcal, Carbohydrates 5g, Protein 11g, Fat 22g, Saturated Fat 7g, Cholesterol 116mg, Sodium 169mg, Potassium 91mg, Fiber 2g, Sugar 1g, Iron 1mg

124. Crispy Everything Bagel Chaffle

Preparation Time: 8 minutes

Cooking Time: 5 minutes

Servings: 2

INGREDIENTS

- 3 tbs parmesan cheese shredded
- 1 tsp everything bagel seasoning

PREPARATION

1. Preheat mini waffle maker.
2. Place the griddle with the parmesan cheese and whisk. About 3 minutes. Please leave it long enough, or let it cool down when it cools down. An important step forward!
3. Sprinkle a teaspoon of everything bagel seasoning over the melted cheese. Once heated, leave the waffle iron open!
4. Unplug the mini waffle maker and urge to cool for a few minutes. This allows the cheese to cool sufficiently to combine and crisp.
5. After cooling for about 2 minutes, it is still dry.
6. Peel warm with a mini spatula (do not use hot cheese in a mini waffle iron; cool completely for crisp chips! These chips pack a powerful crunch that you often miss in keto note: the more cheese you use, the thicker the chips, the less cheese you use, the lighter and crisper the chips!

125. Apple Pie Churro Chaffle Tacos

Preparation Time: 30 minutes

Cooking Time: 30 minutes

Servings: 2

INGREDIENTS

- Chayote apple pie filling
- 1 chayote squash cook, peel, slice
- 1 t kerrygold butter melted
- 2 packets true lemon
- 1/8 tsp tartar cream
- 1/4 cup swallow brown
- 2 tsp ceylon cinnamon powder
- 1/8 teaspoon ginger powder
- 1/8 teaspoon nutmeg
- Cinnamon chaffle
- 2 eggs room temperature
- 1/4 cup mozzarella cheese shredded
- 1 tsp ceylon cinnamon
- 1 t confectionery
- Coconut flower 2 tsp
- 1/8 teaspoon baking powder
- 1 teaspoon of vanilla essence

PREPARATION

1. Blend all ingredients together and mix well in the chayote.
2. Place the mixture in a shallow baking dish and cover with foil. Bake for about 20 minutes.
3. Place 1/4 of the mixture in a food processor or small blender and heat until the consistency of the apple sauce is achieved.
4. Apply the slices to the chayote and mix.
5. Mix shells.

6. Add some sweetener, cinnamon and vanilla.
7. Mix well, guy.
8. Add the remaining ingredients and stir well.
9. Place 3t of the battery in the preheated dash mini griddle.
10. Cook for five minutes.
11. Sprinkle with cinnamon and granular sweetener mixture.
12. To mount, place the chaffles in the taco holders or fold softly to shape.
13. Apply 1/4 of the apple filling to each taco cover.
14. Finish with ice cream or vanilla bean.

126. Pumpkin Chaffle Keto Sugar Cookies

Preparation Time: 10 minutes

Cooking Time: 5 minutes

Servings: 2

INGREDIENTS

For keto sugar cookies

- 1 t butter melted
- 1 t sweetener
- 1 egg yolk
- 1/8 tsp vanilla essence
- 1/8 teaspoon cake batter extract
- 3tbs almond flour
- 1/8 teaspoon baking powder

Icing ingredients

- 1 t sweetener
- 1/4 teaspoon of vanilla essence
- 1-2 teaspoons of water

Sprinkle ingredients

- 1 t granular sweetener mixed with 1 drop of food coloring. Mix well.

DIRECTIONS

1. Stir all ingredients together. Rest for 5 minutes
2. Stir again.
3. Refrigerate for 15 minutes.
4. Put 1/2 of the dough in the pumpkin waffle maker.
5. Cook for 4 minutes.
6. Repeat. Let cool.
7. Add icing and sprinkles as needed.

127. <u>Keto "Apple" Fritter Chaffles</u>

PREPARATION Time: 30 minutes

Cooking Time: 30 minutes

Servings: 5

INGREDIENTS

- "apple" fritter filling ingredients
- 2 cups of diced jicama
- 1/4 cup and 1 tablespoon swerve sweetener blend
- 4 tbsp butter
- 1 teaspoon cinnamon
- 1/8 teaspoon of nutmeg
- Dash clove
- 1/2 teaspoon vanilla
- Lorann oils apple flavor 20 drops

Ingredients for chaffle

- 2 eggs
- 1/2 cup of grated mozzarella cheese

- 1 tablespoon almond flour
- 1 tsp coconut flour
- 1/2 teaspoon baking powder

Glaze drug ingredients

- 1 tablespoon butter
- 2 tsp heavy cream
- 3 cups of powdered sweetener such as swerve confectioners
- 1/4 teaspoon vanilla essence

PREPARATION

1. Keto "berry" fritter filling
2. Cut the jicama and cut into small dice.
3. In a medium-low heat pan, melt the butter and add the diced jicama and the sweetener.
4. Lave it to slowly simmer for 10-20 minutes, looking at it till the jicama is tender, stirring frequently. Avoid using high heat, or the sweetener will easily caramelize and burn. A light amber color should grow and thicken.
5. When the jicama is tender, remove from heat and stir in the spices and flavourings.
6. Keto "apple" fritter chiffle
7. Preheat up to hot waffle iron.
8. Beat all ingredients, except milk, in a medium bowl. Stir the mixture of jicama into the eggs.
9. Put 1 tablespoon of grated cheese on that waffle iron.
10. Spoon 2 tablespoons of the egg / jicama mixture into the waffle iron and finish with another tablespoon of the milk.
11. Open the waffle and cook for 5-7 minutes until well browned and crispy.
12. Remove from the wire rack.
13. Repeat it 3-4 times.
14. Keto "apple" fritter chiffle icing
15. melt butter in a small saucepan and add swerve and heavy cream.

16. Simmer over an average heat for few minutes or until lightly thickened.
17. Stir the vanilla.
18. Drizzle the hot frost over the cuffs. It's going to harden as it cools.

NUTRITION: Calories 186, total Fat 14.3g, cholesterol 108.1mg, sodium 117.7mg, total carbohydrate 8.5g, dietary Fiber 3.4g, sugars 1.5g, Protein 7g, vitamin a 148.2µg, vitamin c 10.5mg

128. Yogurt Keto Chaffle Recipe

Preparation Time: 5 minutes

Cooking Time: 12 minutes

Servings: 3

INGREDIENTS

- 50g (1/2 cup) mozzarella
- 1 egg
- 17g (2 tablespoons) ground almonds
- 1,5 g (1/2 tsp) plantain husk
- 1g baking powder (1/4 teaspoon)
- 20g (1 tablespoon) yogurt

DIRECTIONS

1. Prepare all ingredients and heat the waffle maker.
2. Mince the mozzarella cheese and make the chaffle softer.
3. In a bowl, first mix the eggs with a fork.
4. Add ingredients other than mozzarella and mix appropriately. Once the dough is thoroughly mixed, add the minced mozzarella and mix thoroughly again.
5. Leave for a few minutes to allow physilium to work together.
6. If the waffle maker is not non-stick, spray a little oil

7. To make the chaffle completely crisp, it is recommended to add a little chopped cheese to the bottom of the waffle maker
8. Add a large spoon of dough over the cheese in the middle. Do not add too much. Otherwise, the chaffle will start to spread throughout the manufacturer.
9. Add some shredded mozzarella on top of the dough again and get a crisp feel from both sides of the chaffle
10. Close the lid and cook for about 3-4 minutes.
11. Note: finely chopped cheese works much better
12. Cook until steaming stops for about 3-4 minutes
13. Do not use unshredded cheese because it contains additives and flour to keep the shredded cheese fine.
14. Add shredded cheese to the top and bottom of the chaffle maker to enhance the crispness
15. If the egg feels too eggy for you, replace the whole egg with egg white only
16. Cook for a long time to make it more crispy
17. Do not open the chaffle maker while cooking. Chaffle may be broken. Believe me, i tried it.

129. Basic Chaffle

Preparation Time: 2 minutes

Cooking Time: 6 minutes

Servings: 2

INGREDIENTS

- 1 large egg
- 1/2 cup finely chopped mozzarella cheese

DIRECTIONS

1. Preheat waffle iron.
2. In a small bowl, rub together the one egg and the shredded cheese with a fork.
3. Place half of the mixture equally in the waffle.

4. Cook 3-4 minutes or until golden brown. Remove from the plate to cool. Replace the remaining batter.
5. Notes variations
6. for an egg white cloth, use 2 egg whites or a generous 1/4 cup of egg whites in a carton. Divide and cook exactly as planned.
7. Add 1/8 teaspoon of maple extract to the egg / cheese mixture to a maple waffle waffle.
8. Add 1 tablespoon of finely ground almond flour for the almond waffle. Mix well, guy. Divide and cook exactly as planned.
9. This recipe is for the most friendly flavored chops (with the exception of the maple waffle). You can switch flavors by using other cheeses, extracts and add ins.
10. Other notes:* store in an airtight container in the refrigerator for 3-4 days. Reheat in a toaster oven and toaster.
11. To freeze-wrap each fabric individually in plastic wraps and place it in zip top freezer bags. Store for up to 3 months, to be reheated overnight in the refrigerator or softly thawed in the microwave at low power. Then toast the texture in a toaster oven or toaster.

130. <u>Banana Nut Chaffle</u>

Preparation Time: 5 minutes

Cooking Time: 5 minutes

Servings: 2

INGREDIENTS

- 1 egg
- 1 tablespoon cream cheese, softened, room temperature
- Keto so 1 tbs sugar free cheesecake pudding optional ingredient
- 1/2 cup mozzarella cheese
- 1 tbs fruit sauce
- 1/4 teaspoon of vanilla essence

- 1/4 teaspoon banana extract
- Optional toppings:
- Unsweetened caramel sauce

PREPARATION

1. Average heating mini waffle maker
2. Put the eggs in an average bowl and add all other ingredients to the egg mixture and mix until thoroughly mixed.
3. Half the butter and mix after cook for around 5 minutes until mixture is golden.
4. Remove the completed chaffle and add another portion of the mixture to cook another chaffle.
5. Serve to the top and enjoy warmly
6. Note: let's warm the top with optional ingredients!

NUTRITION: Calories 119, total Fat 7.8g, cholesterol 111mg, sodium 209.1mg, total carbohydrate 2.7g, dietary Fiber 0g, sugars 1.1g, Protein 8.8g, vitamin a 106.7µg, vitamin c 0mg

131. Pumpkin Chaffle With Cream Cheese Frosting

Preparation Time: 5 minutes

Cooking Time: 5 minutes

Servings: 2

INGREDIENTS

- 1 egg
- 1/2 cup mozzarella cheese
- 1/2 tsp pumpkin pie spice
- 1 tbs pumpkin solids without added sugar
- Optional cream cheese frosting ingredients
- 2 tablespoons cream cheese, softened at room temperature
- 2 tbs monkfruit confectioners blend or any favorite keto-friendly sweetener

- 1/2 teaspoon of transparent vanilla essence

PREPARATION

1. Reheat the maker of mini waffles.
2. Whip the egg in a little tub.
3. Add the spice of the cheese, pumpkin pie, and pumpkin.
4. Mix well with each other.
5. Add 1/2 of the mixture to the mini waffle maker and cook until golden brown for at least 3 to 4 minutes.
6. When preparing the chaffle, put all the frosting ingredients from the cream cheese in a bowl and mix until it is smooth and creamy.
7. Attach the frosting of the cream cheese to the hot chaffle and serve immediately.

Notes: Apply the frosting of the cream cheese to the hot chaffle and serve immediately.

132. <u>Sweet Raspberry Chaffle</u>

Preparation Time: 10 minutes

Cooking Time: 6 minutes

Servings: 1

INGREDIENTS

- One large egg
- 1 oz cream cheese
- 2 tablespoons almond flour
- Split 1/3 cup raspberry
- 1 tablespoon confectionery swab
- 1/4 teaspoon baking powder
- 1/2 teaspoon almond extract
- 1 small pinch salt
- 2 tablespoons heavy cream

- 1 teaspoon screenin gold Fiber syrup or other choice sweetener

PREPARATION

1. Preheat dash mini waffle iron.
2. Add egg, cream cheese, almond flour, swab, 2 tablespoons of raspberry, 1/4 teaspoon of almond extract, and baking powder in a blender container and mix until smooth. Place half of the dough in a preheated dash and cook until the light turns off again for about 3 minutes. Carefully transfer to plate with fork and repeat with remaining batter.
3. While the second waffle is cooking, place the remaining heavy cream of the remaining 1/4 teaspoon almond flour and sukrin's gold or your favorite sweetener into a small bowl. Whisk with hand or utensil until cream is soft. When the second waffle is over, add cream and the rest of the raspberry to both waffles.

NUTRITION: Calories 395, total Fat 11.8g, cholesterol 121mg, sodium 221.8mg, total carbohydrate 5.1g, dietary Fiber 1.7g, sugars 1.2g, Protein 11g, vitamin a 133.5µg, vitamin c 7.3mg

133.   Chickfila Copycat Chaffle Sandwich

Preparation Time: 30 minutes

Cooking Time: 8 minutes

Servings: 2

INGREDIENTS

Ingredients for chicken:

- 1 chicken breast
- 4 t of dill pickle juice
- 2 t parmesan cheese powder
- 2 t pork rinds ground

- 1 t flux seed ground
- Salt and pepper
- 2 t butter melted

Ingredients for chaffle sandwich bread:

- 1 egg room temperature
- 1 cup mozzarella cheese
- Stevia glycerite 3-5 drops
- 1/4 teaspoon butter extract

PREPARATION

1. Instructions measures of the chicken: chicken 1/2 inch thick.
2. Cut in half and pick it into a buggy juice from the zipper rock.
3. Seal the buggy and put it for 1 hour to overnight in the refrigerator.
4. Preheat air fryer for 5 minutes at 400* combine parmesan cheese, pork skin, flax seed, and s & p in a tight, shallow bowl.
5. Cut the chicken and remove the pickled juice from the buggy.
6. Sprinkle the chicken in the butter and add to the mixture.
7. In the airfryer tub, roll the parchment paper and gently oil the paper. (i used coconut) put chicken and cook for 7 minutes in the preheated air fryer.
8. Invert a further 7-8 minutes of chicken and airfry. (this may vary depending on the chick size 165
9. Chaffle bread steps: mix everything in a small bowl. Put 1/4 of the mixture in a preheated mini dash waffle iron. Fry for 4 minutes. Go to the office. Repeat x3 assemble the sandwich: put the resting chicken in one chaffle pan and add three dill pickle slices.

134. Chicken Jalapeno Popper Chaffle

Preparation Time: 5 minutes

Cooking Time: 5 minutes

Servings: 2

INGREDIENTS

- 1/2 cup canned chicken breast
- 1/4 cup cheddar cheese
- 1/8 cup parmesan cheese
- 1 egg
- 1 diced jalapeno (raw or pickled)
- 1/8 teaspoon onion powder
- 1/8 teaspoon of garlic powder
- 1 teaspoon of cream cheese

PREPARATION

1. Preheat mini waffle maker.
2. In an average bowl, add all ingredients and stir together till its completely incorporated.
3. Half this mixture and pour a part of the mixture into a mini waffle maker and cook for a minimum of five minutes.
4. Note: optional toppings: sour cream, ranch dressing, hot sauce, coriander, leek, feta cheese, jalapeno!

NUTRITION: Calories 224, total Fat 21.8g, cholesterol 134.6mg, sodium 871mg, total carbohydrate 9.2g, dietary Fiber 2.3g, sugars 4.7g, Protein 18.5g, vitamin a 163.1µg, vitamin c 0mg

135. Crispy Chaffle

Preparation Time: 5 minutes

Cooking Time: 5 minutes

Servings: 2

INGREDIENTS

- 2 eggs
- 1/2 cup parmesan cheese
- Everything except 1 teaspoon bagel
- 1/2 cup mozzarella cheese
- 2 teaspoon almond flour

DIRECTIONS

1. Heat the mini waffle maker for about 30 seconds. Sprinkle the griddle with a range of cheese (i used parmesan and mozzarella cheese), melt and bake for 30 seconds, then add the mixture.
2. In a small bowl, add 2 eggs, 1 cup of cheese, 2 teaspoons of almond flour and bagel seasoning (if you are not a fan, you can skip the seasoning) and whisk.
3. Pour the mixture into a waffle maker so that it does not spill from the bottom.
4. Cook for 4 minutes (the longer the cooking time, the quicker the crisper).
5. This mixture has two chaffles.

NUTRITION: Calories 287, total carbohydrates 6g, Fiber 0g, net carbohydrates 6g, total Fat 20g, Protein 21g

136. <u>Easy Chicken Parmesan Chaffle</u>

Preparation Time: 5 minutes

Cooking Time: 5 minutes

Servings: 2

INGREDIENTS

Ingredients for chaffle

- 1/2 cup of canned chicken breast or remaining shredded chicken

- 1/4 cup cheddar cheese
- 1/8 cup parmesan cheese
- 1 egg
- 1 teaspoon italian seasoning
- 1/8 teaspoon of garlic powder
- 1 teaspoon of cream cheese, room temperature

Topping ingredients

- 2 pieces of provolon cheese
- 1 tablespoon unsweetened pizza sauce

PREPARATION

1. Preheat the manufacturer of mini waffles.
2. In an average bowl, put together all the ingredients and stir thoroughly until fully integrated.
3. Before putting together the mixture add one spoon of cheese (shredded) for few seconds to the waffle iron.
4. This will produce the best crust and making it easier to remove this heavy chaff from the waffle producer when it's done.
5. Add half of the mixture to the mini waffle maker and cook for at least 4 to 5 minutes.
6. Repeat the above moves to cook the second parmesan chicken chaffle.
7. While you slice the provolone cheese add a sugar-free pizza sauce.
8. Tips: after cooking a simple chicken parmesan chaffle, add it to a toaster oven, air fryer, or ninja foodi to make it crispy. Melt the cheese above to make this recipe special. It is worth the effort. You can also pop in the oven for a few minutes until the cheese melts!
9. Totally worth it!

NUTRITION: Calories 304, total Fat 21.8g, cholesterol 134.6mg, sodium 871mg, total carbohydrate 9.2g, dietary Fiber 2.3g, sugars 4.7g, Protein 18.5g, vitamin a 163.1µg, vitamin c 0mg

137.   Avocado Chaffle

Preparation Time: 5 minutes

Cooking Time: 8 minutes

Servings: 1

INGREDIENTS

- Big spray of avocado oil or olive oil/coconut oil large waffle iron
- 2 oz thinly sliced cheese (cheddar or colby work best)
- 1 large egg whisked small waffle iron (single waffle ingredients)
- 1 oz thinly sliced cheese (cheddar or colby work best)
- 1/3 large egg whisked

PREPARATION

1. Sprinkle avocado oil first, then cover the bottom of your hot w. (i cut mine into triangles because i've got a bigger waffle iron) whisk 1 egg together (if you're using a mini waffle iron, use just 1/3 on an egg) and pour over.
2. Place another layer of thin-sliced cheese on top to ensure that you are completely coated.
3. Fry absolutely until the waffle iron can be lifted without the cheese sticking-depending on your waffle iron usually takes around 6-8 minutes.

NUTRITION: Calories 300, Calories from Fat 221, Fat 24.5g38%, saturated Fat 12.3g77%, carbohydrates 2g1%, Protein 19g38%

138.   Original Chaffle

Preparation Time: 5 minutes

Cooking Time: 5 minutes

Servings: 1

INGREDIENTS

- 2 eggs
- 1 cup cheddar cheese

DIRECTIONS

1. Heat mini waffle maker (takes 30 seconds).
2. Whisk 2 eggs and 1 cup cheese in a small bowl.
3. Add the mixture to the waffle maker and spell for 2-3 minutes.
4. This mixture makes two chaffles.

NUTRITION: Calories 168, total carbohydrates 1g, Fiber 0g, net carbohydrates 1g, total Fat 13g, Protein 12g

139. Garlic Bread Chaffle

Preparation Time: 5 minutes

Cooking Time: 6 minutes

Servings: 2

INGREDIENTS

- 1/2 cup mozzarella cheese shredded
- 1 egg
- 1 teaspoon italian seasoning
- 1/2 teaspoon of garlic
- 1 teaspoon cream cheese i like to use flavored cream cheese such as leek, onion, jalapeno, but you can also use plain

Garlic butter topping ingredient

- 1 tablespoon butter

- 1/2 tsp italian seasoning
- 1/2 teaspoon of garlic
- Cheesy bread topping
- 2 tbs mozzarella cheese shredded
- Parsley dash or more italian seasonings

PREPARATION

1. Preheat the oven to 350f.
2. In a small bowl, add all the ingredients of the garlic minced bread until well combined.
3. Divide the mixture in half and cook the first tablespoon for at least 4 minutes. If you like a little crunchy on the outside, i would recommend that you put a tsp of shredded cheese on the waffle maker 30 seconds before adding the ingredients. This is going to make a sweet, crunchy crust that's pretty amazing!
4. After you have cooked both of the garlic bread chops in the waffle maker, move them to the baking sheet.
5. Melt the butter in a separate small bowl in a microwave for about 10 seconds.
6. Apply the seasonings of garlic butter to the butter mixture.
7. Rub the butter mixture over the moist cloves with a basting brush.
8. Sprinkle with a small amount of mozzarella on top of the garlic bread and sprinkle with more italian seasoning.
9. Bake at 350f degrees for 5 minutes. It's just enough time to melt the cheese on top of the cheesy garlic bread chaffle!
10. Serve warm and enjoy a sugar-free marinara sauce such as rao's marinara sauce!
11. Notes: please serve warm and enjoy

NUTRITION: Calories 220, total Fat 10.5g, cholesterol 87.2mg, sodium 87.3mg, total carbohydrate 9.2g, dietary Fiber 1.4g, sugars 1.1g, Protein 4.1g, vitamin a 106.8µg, vitamin c 0mg

140. <u>Cinnamon Sugar (Churro) Chaffle</u>

Preparation Time: 5 minutes

Cooking Time: 7 minutes

Servings: 3

INGREDIENTS

- One large egg
- 3/4 cup mozzarella cheese (shredded)
- 2 tablespoons blanched almond flour (or 2 tsp coconut flour)
- 1/2 tbsp (melted)
- 2 tbsp erythritol
- 1/2 teaspoon of cinnamon
- 1/2 teaspoon of vanilla essence
- 1/2 teaspoon psyllium husk powder (optional, for texture)
- 1/4 teaspoon baking powder (optional)
- 1 tablespoon butter (melted, for toppings)
- Erythritol 1/4 cup (for topping)
- 3/4 teaspoon of cinnamon (for topping)

PREPARATION

1. Preheat the waffle iron for about 5 minutes until hot.
2. If your recipe includes cream cheese, put it in a bowl first. Gently heat in a microwave (15-30 seconds) or double boiler until soft and stir.
3. Stir all remaining ingredients (except toppings, if any).
4. Pour a sufficient amount of chaffle dough into the waffle maker and cover the surface firmly. (for a normal waffle maker, about 1/2 cup, for a mini waffle maker, about 1/4 cup.)
5. Cook for about 3-4 minutes until brown and crisp.
6. Carefully remove the chaffle from the waffle maker and set aside for a crisp noise. (cooling is important for the

texture!) If there is any dough, repeat with the remaining dough.

Nutrition Value: Calories 208, 16g fat, 11g protein, 4g total carbs, 2g pure carbohydrate, Fiber 2g, sugar 0g

141. Pumpkin Spice Chaffle

Preparation Time: 5 minutes

Cooking Time: 5 minutes

Servings: 2

INGREDIENTS

- Pumpkin spice chaffle
- 2 eggs
- 2/3 cup mozzarella cheese
- 3 tablespoons of pumpkin puree
- 2 tsp cinnamon
- 2 teaspoons swab
- 3 teaspoons of almond flour

PREPARATION

1. Heat mini waffle maker instructions (should take 30 seconds).
2. Whisk in one place all the ingredients.
3. Add half of the waffle maker mixture.
4. Cook for 2-3 minutes (the longer you cook the chaffle is going to be the crispier) this blend should make 2 chaffles.
5. Finish with hard (optional) whipped cream.

NUTRITION: Calories 218, total carbohydrates 10g, Fiber 2g, net carbohydrates 6g, sugar alcohol 2g, total Fat 15g, Protein 16g

142. <u>Millet Chaffles</u>

Servings: 6

Preparation Time: 60 minutes

INGREDIENTS

- 100 g butter
- 2 eggs
- 2 tbsp honey
- 200 g millet flour
- 2 msp. Baking powder
- 160 ml milk
- Oil or butter (for greasing)

PREPARATION

For the millet chaffles, mix soft butter with egg and honey until creamy. Add millet, baking powder and liquid and mix to a dough.

Let chaffle dough rise for about 30 minutes.

Grease the chaffle iron, preheat it and gradually bake the dough into chaffles.

To taste z. B. Curd or yoghurt creams, sweet spreads, jam, fruits, whipped cream

Tip: if you want, you can flavor the chaffle batter with orange peel, cinnamon, cocoa powder, vanilla or other spices.

Nutritional Information: 1 Serving Contains (Percentage of Daily Requirement in Percent) Calories 305 kcal Carbohydrates 5 g (net) Roughage 4 g Fat 24 g Protein 17 g

143. Spice Chaffles With Maple Syrup

Servings: 6

Preparation Time: 30 minutes

INGREDIENTS

For the topping:

- Butter (possibly salted)
- Maple syrup
- Some cinnamon
- For the dough:
- 235 g of flour
- 1 tbsp baking powder
- 3 tbsp sugar (brown)
- 2 tsp ginger (ground)
- 1 tsp ground cinnamon
- 1/4 tsp cloves (ground)
- 1/4 tsp salt
- 2 eggs (size l)
- 125 ml rapeseed oil
- 375 ml milk
- 3 tbsp lemon balm
- 2 tbsp maple syrup
- 1 vanilla pod (scraped out marrow)

PREPARATION

1. For the christmas chaffles with maple syrup, first sift the flour and baking powder into a sufficiently large bowl. Add sugar, spices and salt and mix.
2. Mix the eggs, oil, milk, molasses, maple syrup and vanilla pulp and empty to the dry ingredients. Stir until smooth.
3. Heat up the chaffle iron according to the instructions and grease it with oil if necessary. Add the dough and

close the chaffle iron. Bake according to the desired crispiness.

4. Put a piece of butter on each chaffle, pour maple syrup over it and sprinkle with cinnamon. Serve christmas chaffles with maple syrup immediately.

5. Tip: the christmas chaffles with maple syrup also taste good with fresh fruits.

Nutritional Information: 1 serving contains (percentage of daily requirement in percent) Calories138 kcal (21%) Protein2 g (9%) Fat13 g (14%) Carbohydrates 2 g (5%) Added sugar0 g (0%) Roughage8 g (27%)

144. Chaffles With Salmon and Dill Sauce Recipe

Servings: 6

Preparation Time: 30 minutes

INGREDIENTS

- 1 pkg of smoked salmonfor the dill sauce:
- 2 tbsp dille
- 125 g sour cream
- Some saltfor the dough:
- 125 g buckwheat flour
- 125 g wheat flour
- 2 tsp baking powder
- 1 1/2 tsp soda
- 1 pinch of salt
- 2 teaspoons sugar (brown)
- 125 g butter
- 2 eggs (size l)
- 500 ml buttermilk

PREPARATION

1. Prepare the dill sauce for the chaffles with salmon and dill sauce. To do this, finely chop the dille and stir until smooth with the other ingredients. Keep cool until use.
2. Sieve buckwheat flour, wheat flour, baking powder and baking soda. Stir in salt and sugar.
3. Melt the butter and let it cool a little. Mix with eggs and buttermilk and add to the flour mixture.
4. Heat up the chaffle iron according to the instructions and pour in some dough. Close the chaffle iron and bake the chaffle as crispy as you want. Take out and do the same with the rest of the dough.
5. Put a tablespoonful of sauce on each chaffle and drape a slice of salmon on it. Serve chaffles with salmon and dill sauce.
6. Tip: the chaffles with salmon and dill sauce can also be garnished with caviar, for example. They look particularly well presented on a bed of lettuce.

Nutritional Information: 1 serving contains (percentage of daily requirement in percent) Calories223 kcal (28%) Proteino g (0%) Fat25 g (16%) Carbohydrates 0 g (0%) Added sugar0 g (0%) Roughage8 g (27%)

145. <u>Chocolate Caramel Chaffles Recipe</u>

Servings: 6

Preparation Time: 30 minutes

INGREDIENTS

- 60 g chocolate
- 60 g caramel candies (soft)
- 45 g almonds (peeled)
- 235 g of flour
- 1 tbsp baking powder
- 2-3 tbsp sugar (brown)
- 1/4 tsp salt

- 250 ml rapeseed oil
- 375 ml milk
- 2 eggs (size l)
- 1 vanilla pod (scraped out marrow)

PREPARATION

1. For the chocolate-caramel chaffles, roughly chop chocolate, caramel candies and almonds. Set aside a little of the caramel candy and chocolate for the garnish.
2. In a sufficiently large bowl, mix flour with baking powder. Mix in the sugar and salt.
3. Mix the oil, milk, eggs and vanilla pulp and add to the flour mixture. Finally fold in chocolate, caramel and almonds.
4. Heat the chaffle iron according to the instructions and grease if necessary. Empty the dough in and fold the chaffle iron shut. Bake crispy.
5. The chocolate caramel chaffles with the remaining piece of chocolate, caramel and almonds, sprinkle and serve.
6. Tip: whipped cream and fresh fruit go well with the chocolate caramel chaffles. If you like it particularly caramel-like, serve it with caramel sauce.

Nutritional Information: 1 serving contains (percentage of daily requirement in percent) Calories546 kcal (52%) Protein45 g (25%) Fat40 g (24%) Carbohydrates 1 g (4%) Added sugar0 g (0%) Roughage8 g (27%)

146. <u>Hazelnut Chaffles With Maple Syrup and Cranberry Cream</u>

Servings: 3

Preparation Time: 60 minutes

INGREDIENTS

- Oil (for the chaffle mold)
- Chaffle dough:

- 120 g hazelnuts (grated)
- 300 ml milk
- 3 eggs
- 80 g granulated sugar
- 1 pkg of vanilla sugar
- 50 g butter
- 300 g of flour
- 1 pinch of salt
- Maple syrup
- 150 - 200 ml whipped cream
- 1-2 tbsp cranberries (canned)

PREPARATION

1. For the hazelnut chaffles, take the butter out of the fridge in good time and let it soften.
2. Separate the eggs and stir the yolks with butter, crystal and vanilla sugar until frothy.
3. Bring the hazelnuts in the milk to a brief boil, remove from the heat and allow swelling briefly. Beat egg white with a pinch of salt until stiff. Now mix the yolk sprouts with the nuts, stir in the flour and finally subject the snow.
4. Preheat the chaffle iron, spread it with a little oil and bake the mixture into hazelnut chaffles.
5. In the meantime, beat whipped cream and mix with the cranberries. Drizzle the warm hazelnut wafers with maple syrup and serve with cranberry cream

Nutritional Information: 1 serving contains (Percentage of daily requirement in percent) Calories 316 kcal Carbohydrates 5 g Roughage 0 g Fat 24 g Protein 17 g

147. <u>Spicy Olive and Pepperoni Chaffles With Crispy Bacon</u>

Servings: 6

Preparation Time: 30 minutes

INGREDIENTS

- 300 g wheat or wholemeal flour
- 350 ml water (or milk)
- 3 eggs
- 2-3 pods of chili peppers (depending on the desired hotness)
- 150 g olives (black and pitted)
- 30-50 g tomatoes (dried)
- Oregano (dried)
- Pepper salt
- Oil (for chaffle maker)
- Set:
- 150 g bacon cubes
- Oil or lard (for frying)
- Herbs at will (freshly chopped)

PREPARATION

1. For the savory olive and pepperoni chaffles, first cut the pitted olives and the drained dried tomatoes into small cubes, cut the pitted peppers very finely. Place in a bowl and mix with the flour. Do not season too much with salt, pepper and oregano.
2. Stir in the eggs, water or milk slowly and process everything into a viscous dough. If necessary, it is best to let it stand briefly or add some flour. Season again.
3. Preheat the chaffle iron, grease it with a little oil and bake crispy chaffles from the mixture. Meanwhile fry the bacon cubes in a little hot lard or oil until crispy. Arrange baked chaffles on preheated plates, sprinkle with the crispy bacon cubes and drizzle the Fat over them to taste. Garnish with freshly chopped herbs and apply.
4. Tip: the savory olive and pepperoni chaffles can also be sprinkled with a little grated parmesan.

Nutritional Information: 1 serving contains (percentage of daily requirement in percent) Calories546 k Cal (52%) Protein45 g (25%) Fat40 g (24%) Carbohydrates 1 g (4%) Added sugar0 g (0%) Roughage8 g (27%)

148. Cinnamon Chaffles With Fresh Berries

Servings: 6

Preparation Time: 30 minutes

INGREDIENTS

- 250 ml milk
- 400 g of flour
- 4 eggs
- 50 g butter
- 3-4 tbsp granulated sugar
- 1 pkg of vanilla sugar (or scraped-out pulp from 1 vanilla bean)
- 2 tsp cinnamon
- Cinnamon and sugar (for sprinkling)
- Oil (for the mold)
- Set:
- 1 cup (s) of fresh berries (raspberries, blackberries, strawberries)
- 150-200 ml cream (whipped)
- Icing sugar (to taste)
- 1 shot of rum (or grand manner)

PREPARATION

1. First prepare the dough for the cinnamon chaffles with fresh berries. To do this, beat the eggs in a bowl and beat them with vanilla sugar or scraped out marrow and sugar until they are really frothy. Mix the flour with the cinnamon, slowly melts the butter.
2. Stir in the milk under the egg mixture, add the flour and melted butter and stir into a rather thick dough. (if necessary, stir in a little more flour.)
3. Mix the selected berries with icing sugar, stir in a dash of rum or grand marnier and let it steep.
4. Preheat the chaffle iron, spread it with a little oil (butter burns too quickly!) And pour in a little mass each time.

Bake to golden yellow chaffles. Arrange while still warm on plates and sprinkle with cinnamon and sugar. Place the marinated berries next to or on the chaffles and garnish with whipped cream.

5. Tip: the cinnamon chaffles also taste particularly fine garnished with ice cream and chocolate sauce.

Nutritional Information: 6 chaffles contains (percentage of daily requirement in percent) Calories170 kcal (21%) Protein45 g (25%) Fat14 g (18%) Carbohydrates 2 g (4%) Added sugar0 g (0%) Roughage8 g (27%)

149.   Apple Chaffles Recipe

Servings: 4

Preparation Time: 30 minutes

INGREDIENTS

- 200 g butter
- 50 g of sugar
- 1 shot of lemon juice
- 3 eggs
- 200 g of flour
- 1 tsp baking powder
- 125 ml water (lukewarm)
- 1/2 tsp cinnamon
- 50 g almonds (chopped)
- 250 g apples

PREPARATION

1. For the apple chaffles, first peel the apples and cut them into small cubes or grate them roughly.
2. Mix the butter with sugar and lemon juice. Gradually stir in the eggs. Mix the flour with the baking powder and stir in as well. Mix with the water to smooth dough and then add the cinnamon and almonds.

3. Lift the apples under the dough and bake beautiful golden-brown apple chaffles from the dough in a greased chaffleiron.
4. Tip: whipped cream mixed with cinnamon goes well with the apple chaffles .

NUTRITION: Per serving 464 kcal Carbohydrates: 6 g Protein: 47 g Fat: 18 g

150. <u>Gingerbread Chaffles Recipe</u>

Servings: 4chaffles,

Preparation Time: 60 minutes

INGREDIENTS

- 250 g butter
- 1 tbsp orange peel
- 1 tbsp lemon zest
- Gingerbread spice (to taste)
- 4 eggs
- 250 g flour
- 1 tsp baking powder
- 150 g honey (liquid)
- 100 g flaked almonds
- 100 g cooked chocolate

PREPARATION

1. Beat the butter with the aromatics and the eggs until creamy.
2. Mix the flour with the gingerbread spice and baking powder.
3. Sieve onto the dough and fold.
4. Then add the honey and stir to a smooth dough.
5. Add 50 g of the almond leaves and bake chaffles in the greased chaffle iron.
6. Let the cooking chocolate melt in a water bath and brush the gingerbread chaffles with it on the edges.

7. Sprinkle the remaining almond kernels over the gingerbread chaffles

Tip: instead of the gingerbread spice, the recipe can also be prepared with speculoos.

NUTRITION: 347 Kcal per piece Carbohydrates: 2 g Protein: 28 g Fat: 19 g

151. Eggnog Chaffles With Cherry Compote

Servings: 10

Preparation Time: 60 minutes

INGREDIENTS

- 200 g butter (soft)
- 100 g corn starch
- 150 g of sugar
- 2 pkg of vanilla sugar
- 3 eggs
- 150 ml eggnog
- 150 g flour

For the cherries:

- 720 ml cherries (or sour cherries, pickled, in a glass)
- 100 ml port wine
- 2 tsp cornstarch (heaped)
- 1 tsp fresh spice (ground)
- 3 tbsp honey

PREPARATION

1. For the egg liqueur chaffles with cherry compote, first pour off the cherries and collect the juice. Bring 200 ml of juice to the boil with the wine. Mix the cornstarch and new spice with 5 tablespoons of juice, stir into the juice

and bring to the boil. Take off the stove. Add cherries and honey.

2. Whisk the cornstarch, butter, sugar and vanilla sugar until creamy. Add eggs and eggnog in turn. Fold in the flour. Preheat the chaffle iron, brush with oil and bake the chaffles in portions.

3. Serve eggnog chaffles with cherry compote.

4. Tip: eggnog chaffles with cherry compote taste wonderful at easter brunch, for example. If you want to prepare the eggnog yourself, you will find the right recipe here.

NUTRITION: Per serving 924 kcal Carbohydrates: 4 g Protein: 37 g Fat: 49 g

152. Espresso and Pine Nut Chaffles

Servings: 7

Preparation Time: 60 minutes

INGREDIENTS

- 50 g pine nuts
- 2 tsp espresso beans
- 125 g butter (soft)
- 100 g of sugar
- 1 pkg.bourbon vanilla sugar
- 3 eggs (size m)
- 250 g wheat flour (type w480)
- 1 tsp baking powder
- 75 g whipped cream
- 1/8 espresso (freshly brewed, cooled)
- 1 pinch of salt
- Fat (for chaffle iron)

PREPARATION

1. For the espresso pine nut chaffles, roast the pine nuts in a pan without Fat until golden brown and let them cool slightly. Finely chop the espresso beans with a sharp knife.
2. Beat butter, 50 g sugar and vanilla sugar until fluffy. Separate the eggs. Stir in the egg yolks under the butter-sugar cream. Mix the flour, baking powder and pine nuts and alternately stir in with whipped cream, espresso and espresso beans.
3. Beat the egg whites with salt and other sugar until thick and creamy and fold in.
4. Preheat the chaffle iron, thinly grease the baking surfaces. Place about 2 tablespoons of dough in the middle of the lower baking surface and close the chaffle iron. Bake the chaffle in about 2 minutes until it is crispy and light brown.
5. The espresso and pine nut chaffles remove, place on a wire rack and proceed with the remaining dough the same way.
6. Tip: for a variant with chocolate, make chocolate chaffle hearts: chop 150 g of dark chocolate coating and melt over the hot water bath. Dip the cooled chaffles into individual parts of the heart and tip into the warm chocolate coating. Place the chaffles on a wire rack and let the chocolate dry.

NUTRITION: Per serving 321 kcal Carbohydrates: 4 g Protein: 35 g Fat: 14 g

153. Hot Dog Chaffles Recipe

Servings: 6
Preparation Time: 60 minutes

INGREDIENTS
For the cucumber relish:

- 1/2 cucumber

- 1 onion (small)
- 100 ml white wine vinegar
- 35 g of sugar
- Salt
- Pepper (freshly ground)

For the chaffles:

- 2 eggs
- 400 ml buttermilk
- 50 ml oil (neutral)
- 300 g wheat flour (type 405)
- 1 tsp baking powder
- 40 g fried onions
- Salt
- Pepper (freshly ground)

For the mayonnaise:

- 1 egg yolk
- 125 ml rapeseed oil
- 1 tsp mustard (coarse)
- 1 pinch of cayenne pepper
- 1 dash of worcestershire sauce
- Salt

To serve:

- 6 hot dog sausages
- Ketchup (at will)
- Roasted onion

PREPARATION

1. For the hot dog chaffles, wash the cucumber for the cucumber relish and halve lengthways. Scrape out the core and cut the cucumber halves lengthways into strips, then crosswise into cubes. Peel the onion and chop finely.

2. Put the cucumber and onion cubes with vinegar and sugar in a bowl, season to taste with salt and pepper and let it steep.

3. For the chaffles, stir in the eggs, buttermilk and oil until smooth. Add flour and baking powder and season with salt and some pepper. Mix into a smooth dough and fold in the fried onions. Bake in portions in the preheated chaffle iron and let the chaffles cool on a wire rack.

4. For the mayonnaise, put the egg yolk with oil and mustard in a mixing beaker. With the hand blender set up a firm mayonnaise. Season it with salt, cayenne pepper and worcestershire sauce.

5. Heat the sausages in hot water. Place the chaffles on plates and place a sausage on each. Top with cucumber relish and fried onions. Pour mayonnaise and ketchup over the hot dog chaffles as desired.

Tip: The hot dog chaffles are particularly suitable for Preparation in a belgian chaffle iron.

NUTRITION: 332 kcal Carbohydrates: 7 g Protein: 42 g Fat: 28 g

154. Zucchini Chaffles Recipe

Servings: 4

Preparation Time: 30 minutes

INGREDIENTS

- 1000 g zucchini
- 1 onion
- 3 eggs
- 1/2 tsp lemon myrtle
- 200 g wheat flour (type 405)
- 1 tsp baking powder
- 50 g oatmeal (delicate flowers)
- 100 g feta
- 1/2 bunch of dill

- Salt
- Pepper (black, freshly ground)
- Rapeseed oil (for sweating)

PREPARATION

1. For the zucchini chaffles, wash and clean the zucchini first. Use a vegetable grater to cut into strips and place in a sieve or punch. Sprinkle 1 tsp salt over it and fold in a little. Let stand for 30 minutes until the water comes out of the zucchini.
2. In the meantime, peel and dice the onion and sauté until translucent in a little rapeseed oil. Set aside and let cool.
3. Beat the eggs with lemon myrtle, salt and pepper. Add flour with baking powder and stir in. Also stir in the oatmeal. Crumble the feta. Wash the dill, shake dry, chop finely and fold in with the zucchini strips and the onion cubes.
4. Heat the chaffle iron, pour the dough in portions and bake until golden brown. The chaffles zucchini let cool on a wire rack.

Tip: the zucchini chaffles are particularly suitable for an american or belgian chaffle iron.

NUTRITION: Per serving 286 kcal Carbohydrates: 7 g Protein: 34 g Fat: 41 g

155. Mac'n'cheese Chaffles Recipe

Servings: 6

Preparation Time: 45 minutes

INGREDIENTS

- 500 g maccheroni (short or croissant noodles)
- 200 g bacon (streaky)
- 2 onions
- 60 g butter

- 40 g wheat flour (type 405)
- 500 ml milk
- 1 tsp mustard
- 1 pinch of cayenne pepper
- 400 g cheddar (or another cheese)
- 2 eggs
- 70 g panko (or breadcrumbs)
- Nutmeg (freshly grated)
- Salt
- Pepper (freshly ground)
- Oil (for frying)

PREPARATION

1. For the mac'n'cheese chaffles, first cook the pasta al dente in salt water, drain, quench with cold water and drain well. Put back in the saucepan.
2. Cut the bacon into fine strips and pour out a little oil in a pan over medium heat. Peel and dice the onions and add to the bacon. Braise until glazed for a few minutes, then set aside.
3. Melt butter in a saucepan over medium heat. Add flour and simmer for 1 minute. Add milk while stirring constantly. Season it with mustard, nutmeg, cayenne and pepper. Approximately simmer for 5 minutes, stirring constantly.
4. Grate the cheese and stir into the sauce until it is smooth and creamy. Add the bacon and onions and season with a little salt. Add the sauce to the pasta and stir well.
5. Mix one and panko into the pasta and let it steep for 10 minutes. Bake the dough in portions in a preheated chaffle iron until golden brown. Take out and let the mac'n'cheese chaffles cool on a wire rack.

Tip: The mac'n'cheese chaffles are particularly suitable for Preparation in an american or belgian chaffle iron.

NUTRITION: Per serving 325 kcal Carbohydrates: 6 g Protein: 39 g Fat: 32 g

156. Chaffles With Chicken Salad and Tangerines

Servings: 6

Preparation Time: 60 minutes

INGREDIENTS

For the sweet & salty chaffle batter:

- 2 eggs
- 125 g butter
- 250 ml milk
- 12 g germ (fresh)
- 1/2 tsp salt
- 60 g of sugar
- 400 g of flour
- 200 ml mineral water (carbonated)
- 1 pinch of salt
- Vegetable oil (for greasing the chaffle iron)
- For the chicken salad:
- 200 mushrooms (white)
- Salt
- 2 chicken breast fillet (without skin)
- 2 tbsp coconut oil
- Pepper (freshly ground)
- 4 eggs (hard-boiled)
- 100 g mayonnaise
- 100 g of yogurt
- 1 bunch of chives (finely chopped)
- 1 bunch of parsley (finely chopped)
- 4 gherkin (finely diced)
- Sugar
- 1 can (s) of mandarins (175 g drained weight)
- 2 tablespoons of sugar

PREPARATION

1. For the chaffles with chicken salad and mandarins, first make the chaffle batter.
2. Separate the eggs for the sweet & salty chaffle batter. Melt the butter in a saucepan, add the milk and heat it lukewarm. Not warmer! Crumble the yeast into a mixing bowl, pour in the milk mixture and dissolve the yeast while stirring. Add egg yolks, salt, sugar, flour and mineral water and mix everything into smooth dough.
3. Beat the egg whites and 1 pinch of salt with the hand mixer to firm egg whites. Carefully lift the egg whites under the chaffle batter. Let the dough rest in a warm place for 20 minutes.
4. For the chicken salad, cut the mushrooms into slices, salt and fry in a pan without oil until the water comes out and has evaporated. Put on a plate and let cool.
5. Cut the chicken breast fillets into 1½ cm pieces. Heat the oil in the pan and fry the chicken pieces until golden brown until cooked through. Remove from the pan, season with salt and pepper and let cool.
6. Peel the eggs and dice very small. Mix in a bowl with the mayonnaise and yoghurt. Add chives, parsley and pickled cucumbers and season with sugar, salt and pepper. Fold in the chicken pieces and mushrooms.
7. Drain the mandarins in a sieve, collecting the liquid. Set aside a few mandarin wedges for decoration, carefully fold the rest under the salad. Season again with salt and pepper and, depending on how "sweet" you like it, add some of the collected mandarin juice.
8. Grease the chaffle iron and bake the chaffles. Fill the chaffles with chicken salad and garnish with the covered wedges of orange.

Tip: Orange syrup gives the chaffles with chicken salad and mandarins an additional fruit aroma.

NUTRITION: 284 kcal per strip Carbohydrates: 7 g Protein: 33 g Fat: 22 g

157.   Chaffles With Crispy Chicken and Banana

Servings: 4

Preparation Time: 60 minutes

INGREDIENTS

For the sweet & salty chaffle batter:

- 2 eggs
- 125 g butter
- 250 ml milk
- 12 g germ (fresh)
- 1/2 tsp salt
- 60 g of sugar
- 400 g of flour
- 200 ml mineral water (carbonated)
- 1 pinch of salt
- Vegetable oil (for greasing the chaffle iron)

For the crispy chicken:

- 600 g chicken breast fillets (cut into 2 cm cubes)
- 1/2 tsp barbecue spice mix
- 2 eggs
- Salt
- 6 tablespoons of flour
- 1/2 pkg. Cornflakes
- 6 tablespoons of rapeseed oil

For the grilled banana:

- 2 bananas
- 2 tbsp butter
- For the garnish:
- 4 tbsp maple syrup
- 1 pinch of sea salt
- Barbecue sauce (at will)

PREPARATION

1. For the chaffles with crispy chicken and banana, first prepare the chaffle batter.

2. Separate the eggs for the sweet and salty chaffle batter. Melt the butter in a saucepan, add the milk and heat it lukewarm. Not warmer! Crumble the yeast into a mixing bowl, pour in the milk mixture and dissolve the yeast while stirring. Add egg yolks, salt, sugar, flour and mineral water and mix everything into smooth dough.

3. Beat the egg whites and 1 pinch of salt with the hand mixer to firm egg whites. Carefully lift the egg whites under the chaffle batter. Let the dough rest in a warm place for 20 minutes. Prepare the chilli while the chaffle batter is resting.

4. For the crispy chicken preheat the oven to 150 ° c circulating air. Place baking paper on a baking sheet. Season the chicken cubes with the barbecue mixture. Beat the eggs in a deep plate and whisk with a pinch of salt. Put the flour in a second-deep plate. Put the cornflakes in a freezer bag and grind them roughly with your hands; there should still be small pieces. Place the cornflakes crumbs in a deep plate as well. Now turn the chicken pieces one after the other in the flour, then pull them through the egg and then cover them completely with the cornflakes. Press on the breading a little. Heat the rapeseed oil in a coated pan and fry the chicken pieces all over for about 5 minutes over medium heat. Make sure that the breading does not become too dark. Remove from the pan and keep warm on the baking sheet in the oven.

5. For the grilled banana, peel the bananas and cut in half lengthways. Heat the butter in a coated pan and brown the halves of the banana in it; take the pan off the stove.

6. Grease the chaffle iron, bake the chaffles and place on plates. Pour the maple syrup on top, place the banana halves on the chaffles and sprinkle with sea salt. Finally, arrange the crispy chicken pieces on the chaffles and serve the chaffles with crispy chicken and banana.

Tip: If you like, you can garnish the chaffles with crispy chicken and banana with a dash of barbecue sauce.

NUTRITION: Per serving 324 kcal Carbohydrates: 5 g Protein: 48 g Fat: 39 g

158. <u>Eggnog Chaffles With Rhubarb Compote Recipe</u>

Servings: 4

Preparation Time: 60 minutes

INGREDIENTS

For the compote:

- 600 g rhubarb
- 1 stick (s) of cinnamon
- 4 cloves
- 50 g sugar (brown)
- Waterfor the chaffles:
- 200 g butter (soft)
- 150 g of sugar
- 2 pkg of vanilla sugar
- 100 g corn starch
- 150 ml eggnog
- 3 eggs
- 150 g flour

For garnish:

- Some whipped cream
- Icing sugar
- 4 leaves of mint

PREPARATION

1. For the eggnogchaffles with rhubarb compote, first peel the rhubarb for the rhubarb compote and cut off the

ends. Cut into cubes and put in a saucepan with cinnamon, cloves and sugar. Add so much water that the rhubarb is completely covered. Bring to the boil, then turn the temperature back down and let it simmer until the rhubarb is soft. Remove the cinnamon stick and cloves.

2. For the chaffles, beat butter with sugar, vanilla sugar and cornstarch until creamy. Add eggnog and eggs. Finally fold in the flour. Preheat the chaffle iron and brush with oil. Bake the chaffles one after the other.
3. Beat the whipped cream stiffly.
4. Sprinkle egg liqueur chaffles with rhubarb compote with icing sugar and serve with a swab of whipped cream. Serve garnished with mint.
5. Tip: if you want to prepare the egg liqueur for the egg liqueur chaffles with rhubarb compote yourself, you will find the right recipe here.

NUTRITION: Per serving 556 kcal Carbohydrates: 4 g Protein: 41 g Fat: 36 g

159. <u>Chaffles with Baked Beans, Chorizo and Eggs</u>

Servings: 4

Preparation Time: 60 minutes

INGREDIENTS

For the chaffles:

- 3 eggs
- 125 g butter (soft)
- 3 msp. Salt
- 225 g whole wheat flour
- 1 tsp baking powder
- 250 ml milk
- 100 ml mineral water (bubbling)
- Butter (for the chaffle maker)

Optional ingridients

- 250 g chorizo
- 2 pcs. Shallots
- 1 tablespoon of olive oil
- 1 clove (s) of garlic
- 200 g tomatoes (happened)
- 500 g baked beans
- 100 ml vegetable soup
- Salt
- Pepper
- 2 tablespoons of vinegar
- 4-8 eggs

PREPARATION

1. For the chaffles with baked beans, chorizo and eggs, separate the eggs first. Mix the butter and salt until creamy. Add the egg yolks and beat until fluffy. Mix the flour and baking powder and, alternating with the milk, gradually stir into the dough.
2. Add the mineral water. Let it swell for about 30 minutes. Beat the egg whites until stiff and fold in. Bake portions in preheated and buttered chaffle iron and keep them warm in the oven at 60 ° c.
3. Slice the chorizo. Peel and chop the shallots. Fry both in a saucepan in a little oil. Peel and press the garlic. Let it come on briefly, then add tomatoes, beans and soup and bring to the boil. Season it with salt and pepper.
4. Heat a saucepan with salt water. Add the vinegar. Beat the eggs one by one and let them slide into the boiling broth, then pull from the heat and poach the eggs in 4-5 minutes until they are wax-soft. Wash the basil and mint and chop the leaves as you like.
5. Arrange two chaffles with baked beans, chorizo and eggs on plates, season with pepper as desired and serve.

Tip: Garnish the chaffles with baked beans, chorizo and eggs with fresh herbs, such as basil, rosemary, etc. Sprinkle.

NUTRITION: 243 kcal per serving Carbohydrates: 4 g Protein: 33 g Fat: 28 g

160. Chaffle Casserole with Peaches and Flaked Almonds Recipe

Servings: 4

Preparation Time: 60 minutes

INGREDIENTS

- 420 g peach halves (canned)
- 300 g chaffles (ready)
- 4 eggs
- 200 ml milk
- 200 g whipped cream
- 1 pack of custard powder
- 2 tablespoons of sugar
- Butter (for the mold)
- 4 tbsp almond leaves
- Icing sugar (for dusting)

PREPARATION

1. For the chaffle bake with peaches and flaked almonds, drain the peaches in a sieve and cut them into slices. Halve the wafers diagonally to form triangles.
2. Mix the eggs with the milk, whipped cream, pudding powder and sugar. Preheat the oven to 175 ° c top and bottom heat. Grease a large baking dish.
3. Layer the chaffles and peach slices in the baking dish. Pour over the vanilla and egg whipped cream and bake in the preheated oven for 40-50 minutes. If necessary, cover with aluminum foil if the surface tans too much.
4. Roast the flaked almonds until golden in a pan without adding fat. Take the casserole out of the oven. The chaffle pudding with peaches and flaked almonds served dusted with icing sugar.

Tip: The chaffle casserole with peaches and flaked almonds are served with vanilla ice cream a particularly delicious combination.

NUTRITION: 280 kcal per serving Carbohydrates: 4 g Protein: 12 g Fat: 37 g

161. Chaffles With Chocolate Sauce and Mango Cubes

Chaffles with chocolate sauce and mango cubes recipe

Servings: 4

Preparation Time: 60 minutes

INGREDIENTS

- 125 g butter
- 500 g of flour
- 1 tsp baking powder
- 750 ml milk
- 30 g of sugar
- 2 pkg of vanilla sugar
- 4 eggs
- 250 ml whipped cream
- 150 g dark chocolate
- 1 pinch of cinnamon
- 1 mango (ripe)
- Butter (for the chaffle maker)

PREPARATION

1. For the chaffles with chocolate sauce and mango cubes, melt the butter and let it cool.
2. Mix the flour with the baking powder in a bowl. Mix with the milk, salt, sugar, vanilla sugar and eggs. Add the butter and let it swell for about 30 minutes.
3. Heat the whipped cream for the chocolate sauce and stir until smooth with the chopped chocolate and cinnamon.

Peel the mango, cut the pulp from the core and cut into small cubes.

4. To bake, pour a small amount of dough into a preheated, buttered chaffle iron and bake golden brown chaffles. Repeat until the batter is used.

5. Arrange the chaffles on plates with mango pieces and drizzle with the chocolate sauce. The chaffles with chocolate sauce and diced mango serve immediately.

Tip: Serve whipped cream or vanilla ice cream with the chaffles with chocolate sauce and mango cubes.

NUTRITION: Per serving 429 kcal Carbohydrates: 4 g Protein: 27 g Fat: 23 g

162. Fawaffel With Hummus Recipe

Servings: 4

Preparation Time: 60 minutes

INGREDIENTS

- 200 g chickpeas (dried, picked, soaked in water overnight in the refrigerator)
- 1/2 onion (small, roughly chopped)
- 3 cloves of garlic
- 15 g parsley (fresh, smooth, chopped)
- 2 tbsp olive oil (extra virgin)
- 2 tablespoons of flour
- 1 tsp salt
- 1 tsp cumin (ground)
- 1/2 tsp coriander (ground)
- 1/4 tsp baking powder
- 1/4 tsp pepper (black, freshly ground)
- 1/4 tsp cayenne pepper
- Baking spray
- 4 pita bread pocketsfor the hummus:
- 1 can (s) chickpeas (450 g, drained and rinsed)

- 1 clove of garlic (small, pressed)
- Salt
- 60 ml olive oil (extra virgin)
- 60 ml tahina
- 2 tbsp lemon juice (freshly squeezed, more if necessary)

PREPARATION

1. For the fachaffle with hummus, preheat the chaffle iron to medium temperature. Preheat the oven to the lowest setting.
2. Drain the soaked chickpeas and mix with the onion and the garlic in the food processor until they are well chopped but not fully mashed.
3. Add parsley, olive oil, flour, salt, cumin, coriander, baking powder, black pepper and cayenne pepper and puree.
4. Spray both baking surfaces of the chaffle iron with a baking spray. Add approx. 60 ml of the mixture per fachaffle to the chaffle iron, leaving some space between the individual portions so that the fachaffle can spread out.
5. Close the lid and bake for about 5 minutes. Remove the fachaffle from the chaffle iron when it is cooked and browned evenly.
6. Repeat steps 4 and 5 with the rest of the falafel batter.
7. Keep the finished fachaffle warm in the oven.
8. Peel the chickpeas for the hummus: fill a large bowl with water, add the chickpeas and rub them gently so that as many peels as possible come off. The bowls float to the surface, skim there. It is not necessary to peel every single pea that can be left unruly as it is.
9. The chickpeas in a food processor or with a hand blender coarse puree.
10. Add garlic, ¼ tsp salt, olive oil, tahini and lemon juice and puree everything very finely. Season to taste and add more salt or lemon juice if desired. To achieve the desired consistency, always add 1 tablespoon of olive oil or water and fold in with the mixer.
11. Serve the fawaffel with hummus and pita bread.

12. Tip: to be able to serve everything together with this dish, you should finish the hummus while the falafel is cooking in the chaffle iron.
13. Falafels made from chaffle irons are not only much healthier than deep-fried falafel, they are also incredibly tasty, and it is fun to pronounce the wonderful word creation fawaffel.
14. Falafel mix in a bag? It's absolutely fine. Prepare the mixture according to the package instructions. In any case, let them swell for 15–30 minutes so that the dry mass is sufficiently moist. Then cook them in the chaffle maker as described above.
15. Leftover falafel dough can be stored in a sealed tin for several days in the refrigerator. You don't need to bring it to room temperature before baking - just let the falafel cook for 1-2 minutes longer.
16. Leftover hummus can be kept in a closed container in the refrigerator for up to a week.
17. You can replace the tahini with creamy, unsalted peanut butter or leave it out entirely.
18. If you don't want to use tahini or peanut butter, reduce the amount of lemon juice to 1 tbsp.

NUTRITION: 453 kcal per serving Carbohydrates: 4 g Protein: 37 g Fat: 31 g

163.   <u>Blueberry Cinnamon Waffins Recipe</u>

Servings: 16

Preparation Time: 30 minutes

INGREDIENTS

- 240 g of flour
- 55 g of sugar
- 1 tsp cinnamon
- 1/2 tsp salt
- 2 tsp baking powder
- 500 ml milk (room temperature)

- 8 tbsp butter (melted)
- 2 eggs (size l)
- 150 g blueberries (frozen)
- Baking spray

PREPARATION

1. For the blueberry-cinnamon waffins, preheat the chaffle iron to medium temperature.
2. Mix the flour, sugar, cinnamon, salt and baking powder in a medium bowl.
3. Whisk milk, butter and eggs in a large bowl until a well-bonded mass is formed.
4. Add the dry ingredients to the milk mixture and stir into a smooth dough.
5. Gently fold in the blueberries until they are well distributed.
6. Spray both baking surfaces of the chaffle iron with baking spray and pour approx. 60 g of the dough into each baking dish of the device. Close the lid and bake for about 4 minutes until the waffins are golden brown.
7. Remove the waffins from the chaffle iron and let them cool on a wire rack. Repeat step 6 with the rest of the dough.
8. Serve warm blueberry and cinnamon waffins .
9. Tip: leftover dough can be stored in the fridge and used the next day. To do this, follow the steps described above and let the waffins bake for 1 minute longer because of the cold dough.
10. Finished blueberry-cinnamon waffins can be stored well in resealable freezer bags and baked in a chaffle iron at medium temperature (approx. 2 minutes).
11. With a belgian chaffle iron, the waffins become fluffier.

NUTRITION Per serving 524 kcal Carbohydrates: 8 g Protein: 49 g Fat: 25 g

CONCLUSION

From time to time, the phenomenon of food breaks open and unexpected worlds, burning social media like wildfires and sweeping out innocents like tsunamis. What is this natural force?

This is the case for chaffle. Waffle made entirely of cheese and eggs. Sprinkle the minced cheese directly on a hot waffle iron, add some of the beaten eggs, put the cheese on top and leave it to the waffle maker. This chaffle, which was virtually unknown a few weeks ago, sparked YouTube, Facebook, Reddit, Instagram, and Pinterest. In the first two weeks of August, all of Google's key results during this period were posted. Search soared: chaffle mania blossomed so quickly that it was not difficult to pinpoint the originator of the term. The only genius of Chaffle is like a You Tuber named the cat "Keto" Dos. See all original chaffle videos. Dos is delighted with her creation. Although dozens (or hundreds?) Of keto waffle recipes are already scattered around the Internet, the success of chaffle runaway seems to depend on several key factors.

The first is its profound simplicity. Only two ingredients! Most of these other low-carb waffles require expensive alternative starches such as almonds and coconut flour, and often utilize specialized baking ingredients such as xanthan gum and psyllium husk. You can't blame these chefs for trying to make the most sophisticated low carb waffles, but the complexity of such recipes means that they are likely to be used only on special weekends. Made with only one bowl and two pantry staples, the chaffle is easy enough to spin on a whimsical and whimsical basis.

Second, the chaffle community is heroically creative in using chaffle as a bread substitute. A quick search for #chaffle shows that some of the most popular images use chaffle as the base for mini pizzas, hot dog buns, sandwich buns, and more. This emphasis is built in from the start. In the original video, Dos called him a bread substitute, claiming that "the possibilities are endless." Double smash burger.

You cannot miss an ingenious name. This is undoubtedly a contributing factor in the dizziness and abandonment of chaffle head being obsessed with the new obsession. Chaffle was born according to the meme.

CPSIA information can be obtained
at www.ICGtesting.com
Printed in the USA
LVHW011608301020
670160LV00005B/412